Wolfgang Spurzem

Foot Reflexology

Simple Self-Treatment

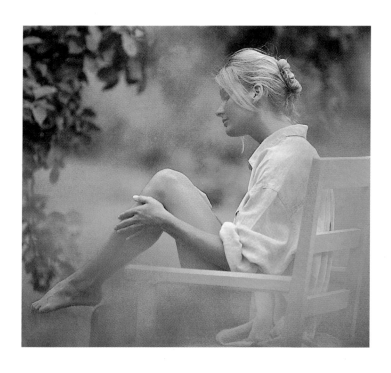

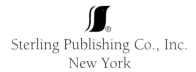

Sterling Publishing Co., Inc.
New York

**Library of Congress
Cataloging-in-Publications Data**

Spurzem, Wolfgang.
   [Fussreflexzonenmassage.
English]
   Foot reflexology / Wolfgang
Spurzem : translated by Annette
Englander.
   p. cm.
   Includes index.
   ISBN 0-8069-9983-7
   1. Reflexology. I. Title.
RM723.R43S6813 1998
615.8'22—dc21   98–19915
                           CIP

10 9 8 7 6 5 4 3 2 1

Published 1998 by Sterling
   Publishing Company, Inc.
   387 Park Avenue South,
   New York, N.Y. 10016
Originally published and © 1996 in
   Germany by Sudwest Verlag
   under the title
   Fussrelexzonenmassage
English translation © 1998 by
   Sterling Publishing Co., Inc.
Distributed in Canada by Sterling
   Publishing
   ℅ Canadian Manda Group,
   One Atlantic Avenue, Suite 105
   Toronto, Ontario, Canada M6K 3E7
Distributed in Great Britain and
   Europe by Cassell PLC
   Wellington House, 125 Strand,
   London WC2R 0BB, England
Distributed in Australia by
   Capricorn Link (Australia) Pty Ltd.
   P.O. Box 6651, Baulkham Hills,
   Business Centre, NSW 2153,
   Australia
*Manufactured in the United States of
   America*
All rights reserved

Sterling ISBN 0-8069-9983-7

Contents

Preface   4

Hand and Foot   6

The Idea of Reflex Zones   6
The Holistic Approach   7
Reflexology   9

Shoes Off, Begin—the Reflex Zones   10

The Feet—A Mirror of the Body   10
The Hand as a Tool   14
The Construction of the Foot   14

The First Massage   16

Massaging Yourself   17
Massaging Someone Else   18
Massage Techniques   18

*Giving your
partner a
massage can
revitalize your
relationship.*

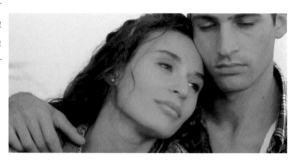

Lesson 1: The Toes 22
Lesson 2: The Ball and the Center of the Foot 29
Lesson 3: The Back of the Foot 35
Lesson 4: The Center of the Foot and the Heel 38
Lesson 5: The Inside and Outside of the Heel 42
Lesson 6: The Joints 43
The Pause—Just As Important As the Work 45

Reflex Zones Used in Treating Problems 46

Eye Problems 46
Intestinal Illnesses 51
Disturbances of the Glands 54
Heart, Circulation, and
Blood Pressure Problems 61
Headaches 66
Stomach Pain and Ulcers 71
Sinus Infections and Sinusitis 73
Back Pain 77
Pain in the Lower Abdomen 82
Toothaches 88
What Not to Treat 91

The Erotic Massage 92

About This Book 95

Index 96

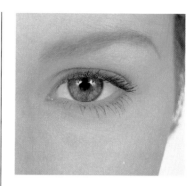

Problems in the area of the teeth are often the cause of headaches and eye pains.

Preface

Do you actually know what your feet look like? No other part of the body does so much or has so much done to it. We squeeze our feet into "straitjackets" and then give them no attention. We only pay attention to our feet when we have corns or blisters or when we step on a jellyfish. Yet, they make all of our movements possible, and they are nature's medicinal treasure, a treasure without equal.

For a long time, people had forgotten about foot reflexology. Yet, this type of massage can provide us with deep relaxation and soothe our pains.

Anyone Who Searches, Finds ...

As a young medical student, I came across an old and dusty book about foot reflexology, written by D. Ingham, an American masseuse. The results described in the book seemed unbelievable to me. Nevertheless, I searched for someone who was knowledgeable about this type of massage. I came across an old beautician and foot specialist who still practiced it. She became my master teacher.

... Deep Relaxation

The education I received from her was the most comfortable education I have ever received because she began with an hour-long massage of both my feet. While massaging, she told me stories from her life, until I finally fell asleep. All of us can have this kind of deep relaxation with foot reflexology.

Old Knowledge

Today, many people believe that, in order to be effective, a healing system must have a complicated theory and complicated techniques, such as computerized tomography, magnetic field photos, and sonograms. We've let machines dominate our understanding of medicine. Some people have gone to the other extreme, insisting that medicine has to be something from the East: Ayurveda, acupuncture, Zen macrobiotics, etc. In our culture, we seem to have forgotten that old medicine exists. Foot reflexology is a very effective technique. It is the fastest and cheapest "X-ray machine" in the world. You only need to take off your shoes! You'll be surprised by what awaits you.

Wolfgang Spurzem

Foot reflexology massage is an excellent way to identify illnesses.

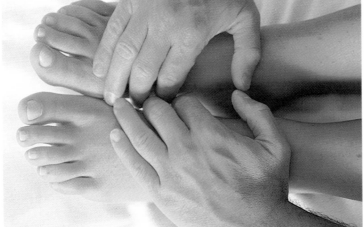

The human feet, one of the wonders of nature, need care and relief.

Hand and Foot

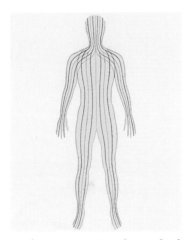

If we use imaginary longitudinal lines to divide the human body, we have ten body zones.

One of the nicest things about foot reflexology massage is that you don't need any kind of tool to do it. Normally, your hands are all you need. Please don't let anyone talk you into buying accessories, such as little sticks, incense, machines, etc. Your hands are sufficient. Also, you'll find plenty of feet to massage. Indeed, you may even wish that you had never told people that you are learning foot reflexology.

Everything is connected to everything, and as it is on the top, so it is on the bottom. This is the basic concept of foot reflexology.

The Idea of Reflex Zones

Dr. William H. Fitzgerald, who studied at the University of Vermont and worked in Boston, London, and Vienna, discovered foot reflexology. I say that he discovered and not invented this because such healing methods cannot be invented; they are found. In this case, we are dealing with experience, and recognizing that according to certain rules, one part of the body always influences or affects another part of the body. This knowledge is as old as mankind. Fitzgerald's interest in the pressure points of the skin surface, and specifically of the pressure points of the feet, goes back to Native American folk medicine and to aspects of Chinese acupuncture. The basic concept of reflexology is that the surface of the feet reflect the entire image of the body and the image of every organ.

Ten Zones

In his book, *Zone Therapy*, Fitzgerald describes the way the body is divided into ten longitudinal zones and the way that all the organs in the body lie within these zones (see the diagram on page 6). Since the zones divide the body into little slices, every part of the foot is a part of one zone. Fitzgerald states that when something irritates one of these ten body zones, this affects an organ which lies in the same zone.

The observation that the hands and feet each contain five lines supports the theory of zones. After all, we can see a pattern in the way the body always grows the same number of fingers. We accept that as normal, but it is also astonishing.

Fitzgerald lived around 1900. That was about one hundred years ago. Quite a few things have changed since then. However, foot reflexology hasn't changed. It is an ancient art, and its consequences can be confusing. Our new understanding of this art is best described by the term "holistic."

They reflect themselves in their respective zones.

The Holistic Approach

The whole is present in each part. That is not a philosophy; it is reality. When you cut off a piece of bread, you have a slice of bread. No one would claim that a slice of bread and the whole loaf are the same. But the holistic theory is that it doesn't matter whether you are looking at the slice or at the whole loaf, you will see everything before you.

"Holistic" is the Greek word for the doctrine of totality. Looking at a hologram provides a good analogy. The laser image of a hologram produces a three-dimensional impression. In a good hologram, you can even look at the object from each side. When you cut off a part of the hologram, the missing piece isn't like a postcard that you cut up. With the hologram, the entire part still exists, but it is somewhat blurred. And the more of the hologram that you cut off, the less focused it becomes. But at no point is even the smallest part of the image missing.

The Part and the Whole

In a way, the body contains a holographic image of itself, meaning that the whole exists in every little part. You can take the foot, the hand, the lower arm, the calf, the ear, the nose, or the eye, and you will always find the image of the whole body in the part.

This knowledge is the basis of old healing systems. It plays an important role in acupuncture, in which we find acupuncture points in the feet, hands, nose, ear, etc. Thus, the concept is not new. What is new is that we are beginning to understand the connections. We begin to see that stimulating a certain point can always produce effects on another part.

The hologram is an image made up of vibrations produced by light waves. Obviously, an image of vibrations also exists in the body, and this creates the inner connections of the cells. That's why five fingers always grow on each hand, and that's why the body also knows when a wound has healed.

> You can use foot reflexology on the entire body, but it should be done on the feet and hands. The principle of the massage is that you can affect inner organs by stimulating the respective outer points.

Reflexology—As It Is on the Outside, So It Is on the Inside

A simpler way to deal with these wonders of nature is not to worry exactly how they function. You can simply rely on experience. Because experience tells you that from the outside, you can influence the inside, and that you can "see" the inside from the outside. In the same way, you can affect all other parts of the body by affecting the feet.

Experience teaches us that we can determine what is wrong with us. That's because foot reflexology does more than treat ailments; it is also a way to find out what the problem is. We only need to know the zones. With that knowledge, we can discover for ourselves what parts of our bodies are disturbed.

Ideal Supplement for Diagnosis

Sometimes, I use foot reflexology in my practice. For example, when I'm not sure what is causing a patient's high blood pressure, I can quickly isolate the zone that is the cause of the problem.

Another example is headaches, which can have many causes ranging from simple tension to a brain tumor. But headaches can also have completely different causes. Sometimes, the teeth, the tonsils, the sinuses, or even tension in the shoulder muscles can cause a headache. You will get an overview of this in the following chapter.

Foot reflexology has a lot to do with experience. The longer you massage yourself or others, the more sensitive you are to the characteristics of the foot.

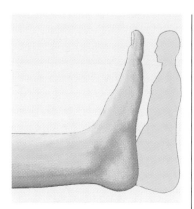

The foot reflects a person who is sitting.

Shoes Off, Begin— the Reflex Zones

Compare the foot to a map. First, let's look at the whole foot. Remember, when we talked about holograms, we said that the foot has a vibration. When you look at the foot from the side, its curves correspond to the curves of your spine.

The Feet—A Mirror of the Body

➤ The heel corresponds to the lower organs.
➤ The toes reflect the head.
➤ Everything between the head and the lower organs is between the heel and the toes.

That's how simple it is. If we want to know where the image of an organ is in the foot, we have to imagine the ten zones. A line leads through every toe. If we hold the feet next to each other and look at them from below, we see that everything that is in the middle of the body lies on the lines of the big toe, and everything that lies at the sides, lies on the lines of the little toe.

In the same way, the left foot reflects the left side of the body, and the right foot reflects the right side of the body.

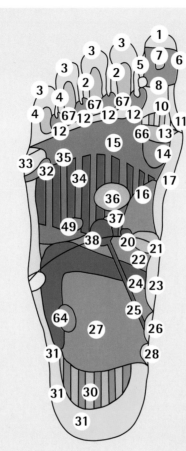
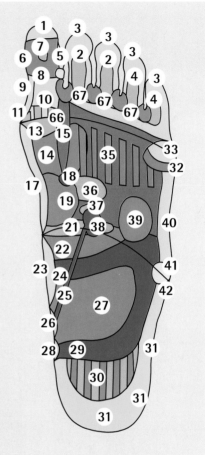

1 Top of the skull
2 Eye
3 Forehead, maxil-
  lary sinus, teeth
4 Ear, tonsils, later-
  al lymph channels
5 Temples, jaw
6 Cerebrum
7 Pituitary gland
8 Cerebellum
9 Base of the skull
10 Neck
11 Spine, cervical
   region
12 Upper lymph paths
13 Thyroid, neck
14 Heart
15 Pharynx, esopha-
   gus, bronchia
16 Stomach, right
17 Spine, thoracic
   region
18 Entrance to the
   stomach
19 Stomach and liver,
   left
20 Stomach, exit
21 Pancreas
22 Duodenum

23 Spine, lumbar
   region
24 Transverse colon
25 Ureter
26 Sacrum
27 Small intestine
28 Coccyx
29 Rectum, anus
30 Pelvic area

31 Pelvic area
32 Lymphatic ganglion
33 Shoulder joint
34 Liver
35 Lung
36 Solar plexus,
   diaphragm
37 Adrenal glands
38 Kidney

39 Spleen
40 Upper arm
41 Elbow
42 Lower edge of the
   ribs, waist
49 Gallbladder
64 Appendix
66 Thymus
67 Tubes

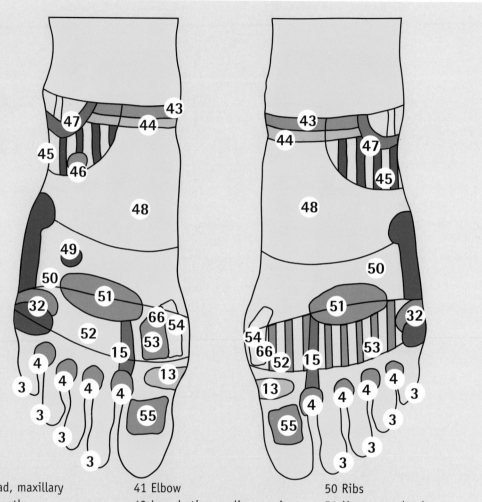

3 Forehead, maxillary
   sinus, teeth
4 Ear, tonsils, lateral lymph
   channels
13 Thyroid, neck
15 Pharynx, esophagus,
    bronchia
32 Lymphatic ganglion

41 Elbow
43 Lymphatic ganglion, groin
44 Groin, fallopian tube
45 Pelvic area, lower abdomen
46 Appendix
47 Hip joint
48 Abdominal wall
49 Gallbladder

50 Ribs
51 Mammary glands
52 Shoulder girdle
53 Heart
54 Breastbone
55 Nose and throat area, oral
    cavity
66 Thymus

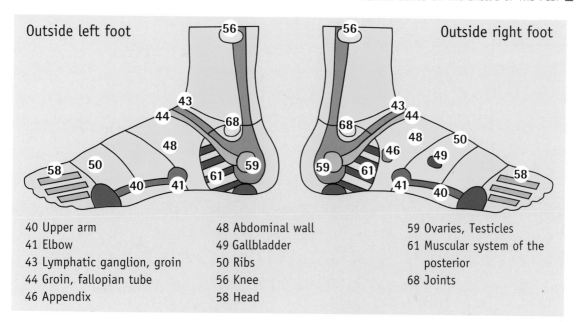

Outside left foot

Outside right foot

40 Upper arm
41 Elbow
43 Lymphatic ganglion, groin
44 Groin, fallopian tube
46 Appendix

48 Abdominal wall
49 Gallbladder
50 Ribs
56 Knee
58 Head

59 Ovaries, Testicles
61 Muscular system of the
   posterior
68 Joints

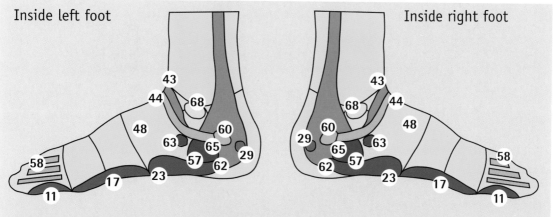

Inside left foot

Inside right foot

11 Spine, cervical region
17 Spine, thoracic region
23 Spine, lumbar region
29 Rectum, anus
43 Lymphatic ganglion, groin

44 Groin, fallopian
   tube
48 Abdominal wall
57 Bladder
58 Head

60 Uterus, prostate, testicles
62 Coccyx
63 Sacrum, ilium
65 Male and female genitalia
68 Joints

The Hand as a Tool

Why We Have Thumbs

Because the hand has a thumb, you can grasp things. In foot reflexology, the thumb is the most important tool. You must learn to feel with your thumbs. When you take your foot into your hand, you can feel the firmness of the sole. When you apply slight pressure, you discover that the foot has soft spots and hard spots. Some spots creak when you press them; others feel spongy. Still others are dry and wrinkled. All of these facts are important.

The most important tool for foot reflexology is the thumb, which grasps and feels.

The Right Feeling

You must learn to knead correctly with the thumb. Be sure you are good to your thumb! Depending on your stamina, foot reflexology can last up to an hour.

The Construction of the Foot

Take time to really look at your foot. Anatomically, the foot corresponds to the hand, except that you cannot

Pay Attention to Your Thumb

➢ Until the muscles and joints of the thumb have strengthened, always begin with short massages. The large thumb joint will be sore if you overexert it.

➢ Only use a little bit of pressure. You don't need to create a hole in the foot. You only need to feel the different layers. To do that, slowly increase the pressure.

spread your big toe apart the way you can the thumb, and you cannot place your big toe on the sole of your foot. We divide the foot into three rough zones.

The Front of the Foot

This area includes the toes and the ball of the foot. It ends at the joint between the center of the foot and the toe joints. Every toe, except the big one, consists of three bones which connect to each other by delicate joints. You can only bend these toes back by stretching the ligaments, and you have to do this with your hand because the toe itself cannot do it. The basic joints of the toes lead to the five bones in the center of the foot. Together with the seven ankle bones, they form the upper surface of the foot (see the diagram on the side).

The Center of the Foot

The spot where the front of the foot becomes the center of the foot is approximately the width of one finger below the groove of the toes. This area represents the transition from the toes to the ball of the foot.

The Heel Region

The second transition, from the center of the foot to the heel region, occurs at the spot where you can feel a small hump on the outside of the foot, precisely in the middle of arch. The inside of the foot and the outside of the ankle indicate the transition of the foot to the lower leg. On the back of the foot, these two regions correspond to each other.
➤ The groove behind the toes towards the back of the foot (front of the foot)
➤ An imaginary line over the back of the foot at the spot of the largest bend of the back of the foot (center of the foot)

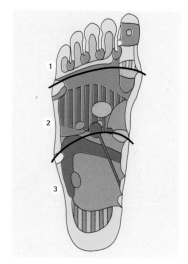

1 Front of the foot;
2 Center of the foot;
3 Heel region

You don't need to learn the exact anatomical term for each bone. You only need to remember the approximate positions of these three areas of the foot.

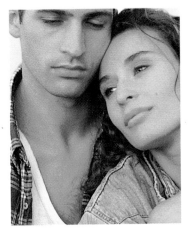

Use gentle pressure with foot reflexology.

In order for foot reflexology to relax you, you must create a quiet and pleasant ambiance.

The First Massage

Before you begin, you need to create the right atmosphere. This is just as important as the massage itself. Make sure that you won't be disturbed for half an hour to an hour. Nothing is worse than jumping up in the middle of a massage because the phone is ringing. Even if you don't jump up, the muscles and nerves of your body react to the telephone. We call that a Pavlovian reflex. Very few people are able to ignore a ringing phone. So, the relaxation is gone because even if you don't pick up the phone, you'll spend several hours asking yourself who might have called.

You should pay attention to a few other things before you begin the massage.

The Room Should Be Pleasantly Warm
This is particularly important if you are massaging someone else and the session lasts a little longer. His or her body will cool rather rapidly. You may want to use a blanket, even in a heated room.

Prepare Yourself Mentally for What You Want to Do
This rule, which is the same one that athletes follow, helps you be more effective.

Cut Your Fingernails Short
Long fingernails can scratch the foot.

What else do you need? Actually, you don't need anything else. But at the end of the massage, you may want a splash of oil. Jojoba oil is perfect for that purpose. You can even mix some with natural fragrances.

Massaging Yourself

Foot reflexology is one of the few massages which you can give yourself. You only need a comfortable armchair or couch and perhaps a pillow.

Place this book next to you so that you can use the overview maps of the zones (see pages 11–13). This way, you can follow the map to know what part you want to concentrate on during the massage.

➤ First, wash your feet, dry them well, and put on one sock.

➤ Place the leg without the sock on the upper thigh of the other leg. The sole of the foot should point up. Sometimes it helps to place a soft pillow under the knee. If you cannot place your leg so that the sole of your foot points up, you might need to lose weight, or you might need to begin a regular exercise program so that you become more flexible.

If you cannot position your legs so that you can massage your feet, try some leg exercises. Until you can massage yourself, let someone else do it for you.

Not too Hard

➤ Older people often have trouble getting their legs into the position described. Please do not try to force the leg into position!

➤ People with varicose veins should not bend their legs for a long time because that will interfere with the flow of blood.

Massaging Someone Else

Massaging someone else and being massaged by that person is much more relaxing than massaging yourself. One of the advantages is that you can stretch out your legs and relax the muscles in your back.

Find a good surface so that your partner can lie down on his or her back. Use a reclining armchair, a bed, or a couch without arms so that your partner's feet can stretch out beyond the end. You should sit so that you have your partner's feet in front of you. Using the floor doesn't work because you would have to bend down too far, and you would tense up and cramp more easily.

Massage Techniques

Begin by grasping the foot (your own or your partner's). Your thumbs should be on the sole of the foot, and your fingers should be on the top of the foot. This gives you a good hand rest, and hand positioning is important in order to massage without producing any tension or cramps.

The Proper Contact

➤ Always maintain good contact with your entire hand! If you hold the foot with only your fingertips, air flows between your hand and the foot. Be sure that the ball of your thumb is on the foot.
➤ This position is important so that the thumb joint has support from below and cannot bend back. Over time, that would damage the thumb. Besides, this position is more comfortable.

Only doctors, masseurs, physical therapists, and similar professionals should charge for massages. Beauticians and manicurists often massage the feet during a cosmetic session, but they do not promise that their massage will heal illnesses or ailments.

➢ In the beginning, pay more attention to your hands than to your feet, even though you are working on your feet. If you don't concentrate on your hands, you will quickly forget the rules mentioned above.

At First, Gently and Aimlessly

Understand your foot by feeling the sole with easy stroking movements of the thumb. You can learn how soft, how warm, and how moist your foot is. At first, stroke the entire foot. Don't concentrate on any area.

Pay Attention to the Toes

Be careful while stroking. The toes need special care.

➢ They are even more sensitive than your thumb joint.
➢ When you press on the toes, you must always support them from behind with your fingers to prevent them from bending back too far.
➢ This is especially important if you are massaging someone else's toes! Normally, the easy stroking movements feel comfortable. But if you come across painful spots, then look at the diagrams of the zones (see pages 11–13). Painful spots hint at disturbances.

Of course, you cannot support all of the zones of the foot, but you need to support as much as possible. Pay particular attention to this support when you are working on the center of the foot.

Begin a Journey of Discovery

Continue to stroke until you feel that you have discovered the underside of your foot. Perhaps a cold foot has become a little bit warmer or a moist one has become a little bit drier.

Once you have finished massaging a foot, keep it warm. You may even want to put your sock back on. Keeping your foot warm will help prolong the flow of energy and the relaxing effect.

In addition, pay some attention to the back of the foot. This area has less padding, and you'll immediately feel the bones and sinews. Use only stroking movements on this area.

Experiment and play with your movements. You cannot do anything wrong if you only stroke lightly.

Later, you can work on the area around the heel, the ankle, and the lower part of the leg. Continue as long as you enjoy it. Work on the other foot the same way.

You will see that you have a completely new relationship with your feet. In principle, you can apply what you have already learned about foot massage to times when your feet are exhausted from walking or standing.

Now We Go Deeper

The actual foot reflexology only begins after you have warmed up the feet the way we have described above. You have two choices on how to begin. You can start at the heel and work to the toes, or you can start at the toes and work to the heel. I prefer to begin at the toes since they represent the head zone even though the toes are the most difficult area to work on. But first, you must use the correct massage grip.

The Caterpillar Technique

For this grip, the massaging hand should be as close as possible to the foot. Bend the last joint of the thumb and exert pressure on the foot (for example, on the big toe)

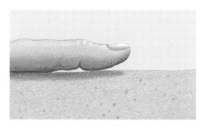
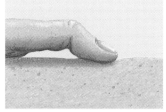
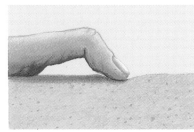
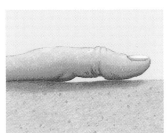

The caterpillar technique involves bending and stretching the thumb. The joint of the thumb maintains constant contact with the foot. However, the pressure changes because of the bending and stretching.

like a caterpillar, moving forward by bending. Now you will notice whether you've cut your fingernails short enough! If not, please do so. Three possibilities can occur during a massage.

➤ Nothing special happens.
➤ You feel pain as if you had not cut your fingernails short enough. If this happens, make sure that you only work with the rounded part of the thumb and not with the fingernail.
➤ The area crunches slightly and feels as if little grains of sand were under the skin. That can hurt.

The last two phenomena are signs of a disturbed zone. Some spots can hurt so much that you can only work in the zone using light strokes. Do not knead painful zones for too long. Work around them.

Keep reminding yourself to work only with your thumb, more precisely, only with the ball of the thumb.

Pleasant Pain - Does It Exist?

Again and again during a massage, I hear people say that it hurts, but that it is also very pleasant. These people aren't masochists. Pleasant pain actually does exist. It indicates that the tissue needs touch and massage in order to reduce the deposits of waste products.

Even though no one has yet determined what the little knots which feel like sand under the skin are, I am sure that they are produced by the metabolism, as is true in the larger muscular system. The fact that these little knots begin to dissolve after several sessions confirms my opinion.

In addition, the pain which you might feel at some of these spots often disappears with time, and the disturbances which caused them disappear at the same time.

You'll find diagrams of the sole of the foot, the back of the foot, and the insides and outsides of the foot. These diagrams always show the left sole of the foot, as if you were looking down on someone else's sole, and the back of the left foot, as if you were looking down on your own foot. All the left reflex points are the reverse on the sole and back of the right foot. When that is not the case, you'll see a diagram of both feet.

Lesson 1: The Toes

Lymph is fluid which bathes the tissues and flows through lymphatic channels and ducts. The sides of the toes represent the flow of lymph to the organs. The undersides of the toes are directly responsible for the organs.

The Big Toe

Begin the massage with the big toe. You can learn a lot from this toe. The zones for many of the important areas of the brain are located in the big toe (see the diagrams on page 23).

The brain and the pituitary gland are located exactly in the middle of the top joint of the toe. Massage the big toe with the caterpillar technique (see page 21). Once you become accustomed to using this technique, you can move to the sides of the toe and massage the lymph zones. There, you "caterpillar" up the outer sides. Later, you can also use slight pinching techniques.

Once you have worked on the big toe below, on the inside, and on the outside, you have kneaded the teeth, brain, cerebellum, pituitary gland, skull, base of the skull, mastoid, neck, the beginning of the spine, and all of the lymph zones.

The mastoid process is a spongelike area of the skull directly behind the ear. It is connected to the ear, and ear infections can spread into the mastoid process.

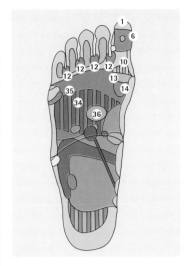

1 skull; 6 brain; 10 neck; 12 upper lymph channels; 13 thyroid and neck; 14 heart; 34 liver; 35 lung; 36 solar plexus, diaphragm, and midriff

A Word About the Spine

The zones for the vertebrae are on the inside of the foot at the transition from the sole of the foot to the inside of the foot (see the diagram at right). Imagine a line which runs from the big toe to the inside of the heel. You can often find disturbed zones in this area.

The transition from the cervical region of the spine to the thoracic region of the spine occurs at the highest point of the ball of the toe. Sometimes this leads to a bend in the big toe, called *Hallux valgus*. This deformity of the toe joint occurs almost exclusively in women who wear the wrong size or the wrong style of shoe. Frequently, the respective neck and spine sections also experience disturbances.

Support the toe joints from behind in order to prevent them from bending back too far.

The Second Toe

The other toes are so important that it is surprising that foot reflexology isn't a required subject in school. For the other toes, pay attention to the sensitive toe joints. Always support the toes from behind with the fingers of the other hand!

Work Upwards from Below

Work upwards from below on the second toe (see the diagram at left). The space between the big toe and the next toe is also very important since that is where the area of the lymph channels begins. Press and pinch the area slightly. Then, work your way up the toe in the usual way, like a small caterpillar, with slight but determined pressure. You will be surprised how many sensitive spots you'll find in that small area. This is the lower part of the eye zone. In cases of tired eyes, farsightedness, and short-sightedness, you should massage this zone daily. Other important points located at toe joints include the teeth and the sinuses.

These organs are frequently the starting point for chronic infections. Therefore, the spots on the foot are often sensitive. Sometimes, you need to work on a spot three or four times before you notice a change, so be sure to give this area enough attention. Don't forget the sides of the toes because the lymph channels run through those areas, too. If you find painful spots in this region again and again, you may need to visit the dentist! Remember that some infections in the mouth can begin without pain.

1 top of the skull; 2 eye; 3 teeth; forehead, and maxillary sinus; 4 ear; 12 lymph channels

The Third and Fourth Toe

Work through the other toes the same way you worked through the first two. Begin with the spaces between the toes and work upwards from below to the tip of the toe. Then, stroke the sides and pinch them slightly with the mounds of your fingers. You'll be dealing with the zones of the eyes, teeth, and sinuses (see the diagram on page 24). The outer sides of these toes are the region of the molars.

Teeth—Not Clearly Defined

In general, the little toe corresponds to the wisdom tooth and the last molar, and the second toe corresponds approximately to the front teeth. But be careful because, in the case of the teeth, the delineation is not totally clear. One region can overlap another. Therefore, you can only indicate the general region in the jaw (plus or minus one tooth). You may find the upper jaw on the back side of the toe and the lower jaw on the underside of the toe (see the diagram on page 27), but that is not guaranteed.

When you feel pain in the tooth region of your toes, see a dentist immediately. Tooth problems can affect many different parts of your body.

An Example from My Practice

I once experienced an especially clear example of how effective foot reflexology can be. My patient had chronic knee problems. The entire tooth area at the third and fourth toe was sore. With an X-ray, the dentist found that the fifth tooth on the right of the lower jaw was infected. The patient had not noticed this because it did not hurt. After the dentist cured the infection, the patient's knee pains also disappeared.

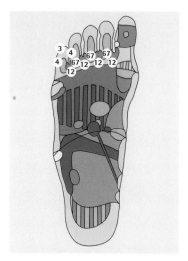

3 forehead and maxillary sinuses;
4 ear and tonsils,
12 lymph channels;
67 eustachian tubes

You can find the entire area of the head in the toes.

The Little Toe

If you remember the concept of the ten zones (see page 7), you will understand that, logically, the ears have to be in this area because everything that is on the outside of the body is also on the outside of the foot. The ear points are located on the lower toe joint and on the top of the toe joint above (see the diagram at left).

This is an area where we frequently find problems which lead to chronic stress and strain. The reason is that many people have had ear infections in childhood. The measles often seems to involve such chronic disturbances. Chronic dizziness, ringing ears, and numbness in the head can then make life miserable. Interestingly, the ear-nose-throat specialist never finds an infection in these cases. Foot reflexology of these points often brings relief. In one case, a new infection of the middle ear occurred. However, after it healed, all of the patient's other symptoms disappeared.

A Small Passage

We should pay special attention to the zone which runs along the lower edge of the eye and the ear zone, from the fifth toe to the second. This is the eustachian tube, the small passage that connects the nose and the inner ear. You can relieve the pressure you feel in your ears when an airplane takes off or lands by swallowing. This helps the eustachian tubes equalize the pressure. When you have a cold, the eustachian tubes can become irritated or infected, causing earaches.

The Backs of the Toes

At the end of the treatment, we deal with the backs of the toes (see the diagram at right). For practical reasons, you'll prefer working on the sides because more pressure points are there than on the top. Also the spaces between the toes are all lymph zones, and they are easy to find from the sides. Between the big toe and the second one, you'll find a soft channel which continues in the direction of the back of the foot. You should work on that next. This is one of the most important lymph zones of the head and neck. You will find pain spots a little deeper here. Cautiously push a little bit deeper with the caterpillar technique.

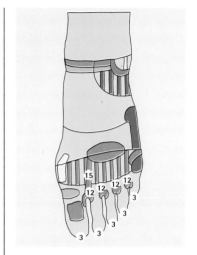

3 forehead and maxillary sinus;
12 lymph zones;
15 pharynx, esophagus, and
bronchia

Pain Creates Tension, and Tension Causes Pain

If you work on these zones on your husband or wife, you will enjoy having him or her "under your thumb!" A little pressure with the thumb at the right spot, and your partner will beg for mercy. Please be nice to each other. Pressure on the pain zones can be very painful. Work carefully around pain zones. If the pain gets stronger with each touch, leave the zone alone. Pain triggers a defensive reaction which produces tension in the blood vessels and muscles. That is the opposite of what you are trying to achieve.

Pain during foot reflexology indicates which zones have problems. The goal of the treatment is not to trigger pain!

When It Tickles

We must talk about another problem which can sometimes occur when you are massaging someone else. Your "victim" may be ticklish. In that case, relaxation is not possible. Men seem to be more ticklish than women, even though we usually think of being ticklish as a female trait. In my opinion, this is often a sign that your partner has little feeling for himself or that he doesn't want to let another person come close to him.

Of course, sometimes people are simply ticklish, and they have no deep psychological problem. Why not try the following for a change:

➤ Place your hands flat on the sole of the foot and the back of the foot. If your partner can tolerate that, then rub his feet with your hands.

➤ If he finds this ticklish, then use some oil to really coat the foot. Often, people perceive this as being more pleasant.

➤ Try a somewhat firmer pressure. See if this is less uncomfortable. Maybe you are simply proceeding too cautiously.

If these measures don't help, then your partner is out of luck.

> When you cannot massage the foot, you can use hand reflexology. Although you can do reflex massages on other body parts, these massages are best left to the experts.

Why Not Take a Hand in Your Hand for a Change

As an alternative, you can massage the hands instead of the feet. You can achieve similar results with the hands. The basic pattern is the same. Simply imagine that the fingers are the toes and the base of the hand is the heel. The position of the zones is about the same.

Lesson 2: The Ball and the Center of the Foot

After you have worked through the head region in the toes, the next region is the chest. These reflex points are less difficult than the ones in the head zones because this part of the foot has no sensitive joints. However, you do need to pay a lot of attention to your thumb since you'll need to apply more pressure in the center of the foot.

Many important organs in the chest are located in the area halfway between the ball of the foot and the heel (see the diagram on page 30). The imaginary line that divides the ball of the foot and the heel corresponds to the navel. According to the concept of the ten zones, we can find all of the organs and their positions in the respective zones. This means that different organs are located on the left and on the right.

The following is a little refresher course in anatomy.

In the Center—The Solar Plexus

Place your thumb approximately on the center of the foot. Here, you hit one of the most sensitive points, the solar plexus. This is one of the most important nerve centers in the abdominal area because it supplies the nerve connections and regulates the blood supply to all the organs of the upper abdominal area. You feel the effects of the solar plexus when you are frightened. You have the feeling that your belly has become empty. A strong push into this nerve center causes breathing problems. In fact, if the push is strong enough, breathing can stop, you don't get any air, and you may even lose consciousness.

Not all of the organs in the body are symmetrical. Certain reflex points are only in one foot—for example, the heart, the liver, and the stomach.

13 thyroid gland; 14 heart;
16 stomach (right);
19 stomach and liver (left);
34 liver; 35 lung;
36 solar plexus and diaphragm

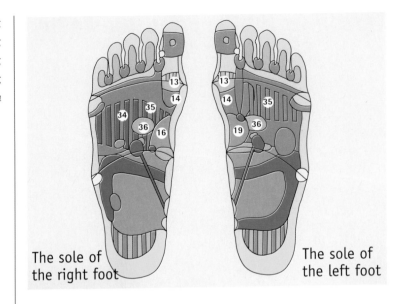

The sole of the right foot

The sole of the left foot

The solar plexus is frequently disturbed. All chronic illnesses of the upper abdominal organs are reflected in the solar plexus point.

When the Breathing Is Disturbed

Our sedentary lifestyle doesn't give the diaphragm enough movement. As a result, breathing is blocked. Relaxed breathing doesn't give the diaphragm a regular inner massage because the organs are pressed together. When you inhale, these organs are like a sponge, and when you exhale, they fill themselves with new blood.

The solar plexus also needs an inner massage. Massage the solar plexus point several times with slightly circulating movements of your thumb. Then, "caterpillar" from the edge of the ball of the foot upwards to the starting point of the big toe.

Notice that foot reflexology of the solar plexus point leads to deeper, more relaxed breathing. That is especially true when the patient is lying down.

There, you come through the areas of the liver, lung, and thyroid on the right and through the heart, lung, and thyroid gland on the left. In this list, you will notice the following:

➤ The heart is on the left and on the right. Also on the right is the liver, in exactly the position which it has in the body.

➤ Some organs overlap in their reflex zones. For example, the liver reaches under the chest and thus affects the lung area, and the heart also lies in the lung area, especially on the left. Therefore, the distinction between the organs is not always easy to determine in the center of the foot.

The Heart

The heart zone is not just in the left foot. The real position of the heart is the center of the chest, reaching into the lung on the left. We look for the heart reflex point directly above the solar plexus. Unfortunately, the overlap with the lung zone is so big that we cannot distinguish from the position of the pain whether the problem is the lung or the heart.

We often find that a pain point in the area of the lung will mirror sensitive spots on the lung area on the right. Frequently, people with lung illnesses have strong, horny growths in the lung zone of their feet. This phenomenon is not often found in people who have illnesses of the heart.

The Lungs

The lungs occupy the largest part of the ball of both the right and left foot. The area covers practically the entire center of the foot.

In case of heart problems, work on the left foot, even though the heart reflex zone is located on both the left and right foot.

12 lymph zone;
15 pharynx; esophagus, and
bronchia; 16 stomach;
18 stomach entrance;
19 stomach and liver;
20 pyloric sphincter;
22 duodenum;
32 shoulder lymphatic ganglion;
33 shoulder joint; 34 liver;
36 solar plexus

The sole of the right foot

The sole of the left foot

In case of a serious ailment in the abdominal area, see a doctor. Do not massage the area if you are at all suspicious! In this area, the pain could be from an organ other than the stomach.

The bronchial tubes are located around the area of the ball of the feet. Foot reflexology can be very helpful in cases of a cough or bronchitis. The ball of the foot actually reflects the neck and the larynx (see the diagram above).

The lung zone merges with the shoulder joint zone at the side of the little toe. Seen from the center line, the shoulder joint lies on the outside of the body.

The Stomach

Because the stomach runs transversely through the two halves of the body, it is reflected on the right and the left, next to the solar plexus (see the diagram above). You can find it on the first zone line, which begins at the big toe. The stomach zone can go up to the inside of the foot, and this zone can be very sensitive. The pyloric sphincter and

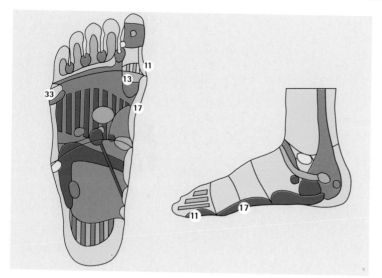

Inside of the foot:

11 neck and spine;

17 chest

Sole of the foot:

11 cervical region of the spine;

13 thyroid gland;

17 thoracic region of the spine,

33 shoulder joint

the duodenum are found on the right foot. The zone reacts in cases of stomach cramps, ulcers, and infections.

Neck and Chest

Since the cervical portion of the spine, which lies at the inner edges of the feet, is frequently disturbed, the zones in the foot may be painful. They lie exactly on the transition from the toe joint to the ball of the foot. Thus, they jut into the larynx area, even though they do so laterally. The area for the larynx and the thyroid gland lies exactly on the ball of each foot. Treat this area for all thyroid problems.

The entire shoulder girdle and all the muscles of the neck and the shoulders are located on the bulges of the toe joints. They are especially soft and fleshy. The area of the lymph glands of the neck and chest are also found there.

Just as with back massages, begin the first few treatments with gentle strokes and little pressure. With the patient's consent, you may use the stronger caterpillar technique.

Working through the Center of the Foot

As we have seen, all of the important organs of the chest and abdominal region are located in the center of the foot. Sections of the spine are also in this area. Proceed with the massage as follows:

➤ After you have worked on the solar plexus, "caterpillar" yourself up to the shoulder zones and work along the toe roots. That way, you'll also pass along the ball of the foot. You should work that thoroughly as well. Work from the tip of the mound to the outside, moving downwards. Use a star-shaped pattern, continuing until you have kneaded all of the sides.

➤ Work on the bulge of the front of the foot from the center upwards.

➤ After that, follow the line below the toe joints from the inside to the outside or vice versa and finally through the shoulder region on the fifth line and the spine on the first line.

➤ For the spine, begin at the center of the inner edge of the foot and work up to the big toe. Work that toe a little bit since the base of the skull and the endings of the muscular system are located there.

You use the caterpillar technique in a star-shaped pattern, working little by little on all parts of the zone, starting in the center and working towards the sides.

The Back of the Foot

Perhaps you've already felt some sensitive spots on the back of the foot while you've been working on the sole of the foot. Additional zones for the jaw and shoulder muscles are located here.

Ideally, you only use a little pressure when you massage the back of the foot. Feel your way along the ankles (compare this to Lesson 3).

Lesson 3: The Back of the Foot

Teeth

We have already addressed the position of the teeth in the previous chapters. However, we want to review them briefly (see the diagram at right).

➢ Big toe: front tooth (1)
➢ Second toe: second and third tooth (2, 3)
➢ Third toe: fourth and fifth tooth (4, 5)
➢ Fourth toe: sixth and seventh tooth (6, 7)
➢ Little toe: wisdom tooth (8)

While the underside of the toes concerns the lower jaw, the back of the foot seems to represent the upper jaw. But that has not yet been sufficiently researched.

The tooth zones lie around each toenail. They can be reached only with relatively pointy pressure with the forefinger. To do this, press the tip of the forefinger into the area between the toe and the nail until you make contact with the bone and skin of the toe. Please avoid bending a toe back too far!

The Jaw and Throat Area

The maxillary sinus zones begin below the toenails in the direction of the center of the foot. They reach up to the toe root. We always treat this zone from the front and side of the toe to the back side. The first joint of the big toe carries the zone for the entire nose and throat area. If you have a runny nose, it is worthwhile working on this zone.

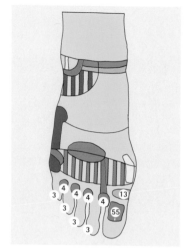

3 teeth 1–8, maxillary sinus;
4 ear, tonsil, and lateral lymph
channels; 13 thyroid gland;
55 nose and jaw

You can treat the zones of the teeth in all cases of chronic toothaches. However, if you feel pain in those points, you should see a dentist.

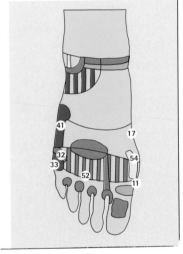

11 cervical portion of the spine;
17 thoracic region of the spine;
32 lymph channel in the shoulder;
33 shoulder joint;
41 elbow and elbow joint;
52 shoulder girdle;
54 breastbone

Lymph Zones and Glands

As you already know, the lymph zones are on the inside and the outside of the toe. We find the tonsils in the web between the big toe and the second toe. The thyroid zone runs up to the back of the foot. The larger the gland, the larger the reflex area. These large glands also seem to run backwards.

The Shoulder Girdle

I want to recommend that you work on the shoulder girdle (see the diagram at left). In today's world, everyone seems to have tensions in this region, and treating it is helpful.

The dividing line between the front of the foot and the center of the foot lies exactly on the toe joint. If you imagine that the shoulders are on the outside of the trunk, then you know that the reflex point must be exactly on the side of the ball of the little toe.

The breastbone represents the bony center line of the chest. Therefore, the zone it belongs to lies on the side of the big toe, exactly on the inner edge. Logically, we would find the shoulder girdle right between these two zones. The shoulder girdle zone represents the front part of the shoulder muscle (from below the collarbone up over the shoulders).

Tennis Elbow—a Tip from My Practice

If you have tennis elbow, you can easily find the zone of the upper arm to the elbow by stroking from the shoulder joint point in the direction of the center of the foot.

The Rib Zones on the Back of the Foot

The rib zones are below the shoulder girdle zone, spread out over the entire width of the back of the foot (see the diagram at right). You can loosen tension in the ribs there, but you must not press too hard because the bone is close to the surface. Too much pressure there will hurt.

The Gallbladder Point

The gallbladder reflex point represents something special on the back of the foot. It lies on the side of the little toe, between the fourth and the fifth line, below the breast gland zone (see the diagram at right). You can only find this point on the right foot because the gallbladder is on the right side of the body.

Bronchial Tubes and Esophagus

Finally, we want to mention again the zone for the esophagus and the bronchial tubes. You can find these at the same spot on the sole of the foot, between the big toe and the second line.

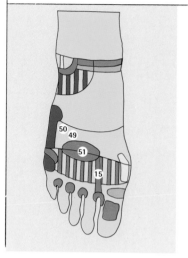

15 pharynx, esophagus, and bronchia; 49 gallbladder; 50 ribs; 51 mammary glands

A Female Massage

For women, you need to pay special attention to the zone that covers the breasts. This zone lies exactly in the middle of the first and second dividing line, in other words, between the front of the foot and the center of the foot. Give this area a careful, easy massage daily for prophylactic purposes.

Here's a tip for times when you have problems with your gallbladder. If you have acute cramping in the area of the gallbladder, applying very strong pressure on the gallbladder point often removes the pain.

Lesson 4: The Center of the Foot and the Heel

Returning to the sole of the foot, we find the zones for the stomach and the lower abdominal organs. Of course, all the organs lie in their respective zones on the foot.

The Kidney and Adrenal Glands

If we slide down about as much as the width of the ball of the thumb from the solar plexus, we come across another very important point. This is the reflex point of the kidney and adrenal glands. The kidney is an important organ because it removes toxins from the body. On the other hand, the adrenal glands have nothing at all to do with

The body produces the most important hormones, adrenaline and cortisone, in the adrenal glands.

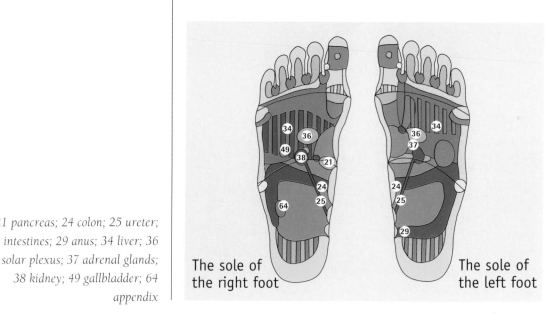

The sole of the right foot

The sole of the left foot

21 pancreas; 24 colon; 25 ureter; 27 intestines; 29 anus; 34 liver; 36 solar plexus; 37 adrenal glands; 38 kidney; 49 gallbladder; 64 appendix

urine formation. These glands, which sit on the kidney, produce hormones.

The reflex points are especially important because the kidneys are often disturbed without our knowing it. You can treat old infections of the urinary tract and chronic pyelitis here. Such chronic ailments are often a medical problem, treated again and again with antibiotics.

When the kidney point is sensitive, this is always a sign that the kidneys are not okay. Since this point also treats the adrenal glands, we can help allergies, infections, and stress because when we are under stress, the adrenal glands are often overactive (see page 59).

The Intestines

Everything below the kidney points, up to the heel, belongs to the reflex zone of the intestines. To begin, we distinguish between the small intestine and the colon and their different zones. The small intestine is responsible for a large part of digestion. The colon thickens the fluid contents of the intestines.

The Colon

The colon, the last part of the intestines, spreads out in the shape of a horseshoe over the belly. It begins in the right groin, goes up towards the liver, goes across the belly to the other side, then runs down again to the left groin, and finally runs to the end of the intestines in the center of the body, where it becomes the anus. We find colon zones on the outer edge of the right foot, just before the heel. From there, the zone runs up the center of the foot (the border of the abdomen) and continues to the inner edge of the foot.

Our intestinal tract always contains fungi and bacteria. Illnesses and antibiotics can destroy these natural inhabitants, leading to an infection in the intestinal tract.

The intestinal zone continues from the inner edge of the left foot to the outer edge. Then, it turns down towards the left heel, where it bends to the inner edge of the left foot. Therefore, most of the colon is on the left foot (see the diagram on page 38).

Hemorrhoids

In case of hemorrhoids, you should treat the end point of the colon.

Appendix

Here's an important spot in the colon zone on the right foot. It lies in the middle between the heel and the abdominal line and is approximately the width of one thumb from the outer edge of the foot. This point, which corresponds to the appendix, lies very deep.

If you have pains in the lower right abdominal area, and you're not sure if the appendix is involved, test this point. Sometimes, if the appendix is inflamed, it is very sensitive to pressure, but you cannot always feel the point. In cases of appendicitis, never rely solely on the reflex point! Always see a doctor.

Hemorrhoids are abnormal expansions of the vessels in the lower intestines. Constipation, diarrhea, and a genetic predisposition are important factors in the formation of hemorrhoids.

Don't Diagnose Yourself!

I have experienced cases in which, after a short period of pain, the appendicitis seemed to have healed itself. Some days later, though, the inflamed appendix was about to burst. Even today, a burst appendix can be very serious.

The Small Intestine

Everything that lies below the arch of the colon involves the small intestine. The small intestine lies curled up in the middle of the abdomen. Thus, the entire rear area of the sole of the foot up to the heel is the zone of the small intestine.

The small intestine is divided into several sections.

The Ureter

The ureter is rather special. Its zone runs in a straight line from the kidney point to the inside of the foot. In cases of chronic kidney and bladder ailments, the part of the zone which is close to the inner edge of the foot can be sensitive to pressure.

The Right Massage

Knead the entire center of the foot and heel area with the thumb using the caterpillar technique. Since the tissue is especially thick, you may apply more force here. Please pay attention to your thumb. Be sure you support it by keeping it nestled close to the sole of the foot.

The farther you work along the sole of the foot towards heel, the more pressure you must apply to get the desired result on the harder spots of the foot.

The Heel

We have almost finished the sole of the foot. Only the heel remains. It is made of such strong tissue that it requires considerable pressure in order to work on it.

The pelvic regions lie on the heel. But only the zones of the pelvic organs end there. The actual zones of the lower abdominal organs are on the inside and outside of the heel.

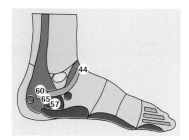

44 groin; 57 bladder; 60 prostate,
testicles, and ovaries; 65 male and
female genitalia

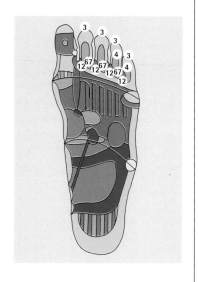

3 forehead and maxillary sinus;
4 ear and tonsils; 12 lymph zones;
67 tubes

Lesson 5: The Inside and Outside of the Heel

The points for the lower abdomen are on the inside and outside of the heels (see the diagram at left). We saw the ureter when we discussed the kidney zone. We know that it runs into the bladder region. The bladder zone is on the inner edge of the heel, directly above the sacrum region. The entire zone, up to the ankle of the foot, is the lower abdomen. We often find spots here which react painfully to pressure, indicating a swelling or a blockage. In cases of poor blood circulation in the pelvic area, the veins are sometimes blocked up to here.

In men, the prostate zone lies directly above the bladder region. In women, the fallopian tube lies above the bladder region. From here, a groin zone winds over the instep. In women, the ovary zone and all its lymphatic ganglions are in this region. The groin zone runs over the instep to the outer edge of the foot, where the zone for the testicle and ovary lies.

The Right Massage

I recommend a somewhat different stroke technique at the inside and outside of the heel. Here, the thumb pressure should be shaped like the figure "8". Lying on its side, the figure "8" is a symbol for eternity. However, the reflex zones do not care about that. They are simply pleased about the highly effective stimulation, which is better than normal pressure. After working on the lower abdominal zone, we go about 2 inches (5 cm) up the lower leg. These zones correspond to the legs.

Lesson 6: The Joints

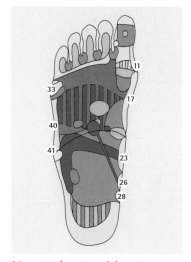

Even though we've already discussed the spine and its small joints, I want to mention them again at this point with all the other joints (see the diagram on the right).

Let's remember that what lies in the middle of the body lies on the inside of the feet, and what lies on the outside of the body lies at the outer edge of the feet.

➤ The reflex zone of the cervical portion of the spine begins at the big toe at about the first toe joint. The next vertebrae are below that in the direction of the heel.

➤ The transition from the cervical region to the thoracic region of the spine is a very sensitive area, located at the ball of the foot.

➤ We look for the transition from the thoracic region of the spine to the lumbar region of the spine at the abdominal line.

➤ Now, we simply go down to the beginning of the heel to reach the sacrum, pelvic bone, and the coccyx.

You need to work on this imaginary line at the inner edge of the foot one more time at the end of each massage. The spine is very important for the proper functioning of the entire nervous system.

11 cervical region of the spine;
17 thoracic region of the spine;
23 lumbar region of the spine;
26 sacrum; 28 coccyx;
33 shoulder joint; 40 upper arm;
41 elbow

Pay special attention to the zone of the spine on the inner edge of the foot. We find the lumbar region of the spine from the abdominal line down to the small of the back. The coccyx is also located down there. These zones are often extremely sensitive.

Shoulder and Arm Area

After you massage the spine, look for the other joint zones and work them as well. The shoulder zone is located at the spot where the little toe joins the foot. The zone extends about the width of one thumb up the back of the foot.

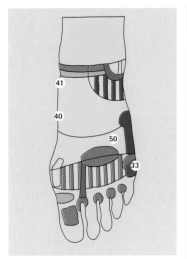

33 shoulder joint; 40 upper arm;
41 elbow; 50 ribs

The zone for the upper arm to the elbow is also at the juncture of the little toe and the foot. It runs up to the middle of the outer edge of the foot, but it is stronger on the back of the foot (see the diagram on the left). On the back of the foot, the area between the ankle bones corresponds to the rib zones.

The Leg Region

We find the upper leg zone in the heel area (see the diagram below). It runs upwards in a straight line above the outer ankle for 1 inch (2.5 cm) or so. The knee is about the width of a hand away from the ankle. On the inside, exactly opposite the knee, is the upper thigh. You should also work on these zones again at the end. Complete the massage by stroking the feet very lightly with both hands. This provides a very pleasant finish.

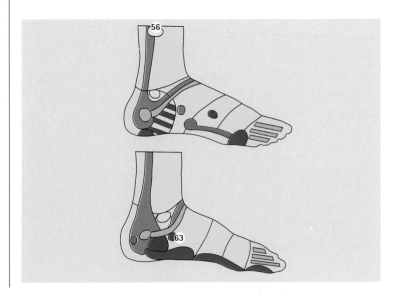

56 knee; 63 ilium

The Pause—Just As Important As the Work

Generally, people should avoid jumping up immediately after the massage to catch up on what they think they've missed during the massage. Urge your patient to have a ten-minute pause or rest period. Wrap the feet up again so that they are nice and warm and cover your patient with a blanket. Now, you've finished the treatment. The interval between two sessions can be one to seven days. In cases involving difficult or acute problems, provide a daily massage. In cases involving chronic problems, once or twice a week is sufficient.

Before We Continue

In the following, I will describe how to treat yourself. Foot reflexology helps every ailment! You can treat every one of your problems and those of your friends and acquaintances. However, you must pay attention to some things.

➢ Never recommend that someone skip or ignore treatments prescribed by a doctor, suggesting foot reflexology instead.

➢ Foot reflexology doesn't replace a doctor's diagnosis. Only a doctor can be sure that the ailment isn't caused by a serious illness which might require intensive medical treatment.

➢ If you are not a doctor or a medical practitioner, you may not accept money for treating a patient. If you do, you may be breaking the law.

You can use foot reflexology simply to relax the feet and the body.

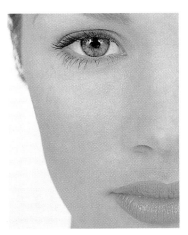

You've reached the first goal. After six lessons, you are ready to use foot reflexology.

Never give a massage in only one zone. In case of specific problems with one organ, don't skip the overall treatment.

Reflex Zones Used in Treating Problems

Eye Problems

Many eye problems, especially chronic ones, respond to foot reflexology. After all, the eye is not just an isolated organ in the head or a mechanical camera; it is part of the entire body, and many other spots influence it.

Glaucoma (increased pressure within the eye)

With the following case, I'm going to illustrate how complicated the circumstances of an eye problem can be and how hard it is to return the eye to good health.

➤ Mr. P. was depressed. The eye doctor explained to him that he was suffering from an especially malicious form of glaucoma. This is a disease in which the pressure in the eye increases so much that the patient may lose sight in the eye. His doctor tried special medicines, but these only lowered the eye pressure slightly. The possibility of an operation became more and more likely. An acquaintance suggested foot reflexology. A doctor taught him to give himself massages.

As we know, the eye zones are on the underside of the second and third toe (see the diagram on page 47) on the left and the right foot. However, rushing to this spot and kneading it in the hopes of producing a cure is not going to be helpful. Even in cases of a serious illness, as described above, the cause can lie somewhere else. Therefore, you should proceed with caution. First, get an idea of what is happening in all the zones by carefully examining and feeling the foot. Then, you can knead all the zones once, briefly. Work on the eye zone last. This will prevent you from drawing the wrong conclusions.

➤ Mr. P. massaged his feet daily. He worked on each foot for about fifteen minutes. At the next checkup, he said, "It's strange. I begin the massage by stroking my feet. Then, I get so tired that I could fall asleep. I don't feel at all like continuing to massage. I don't think I will ever learn how to do it. I don't seem to have any willpower!"

➤ That was not the case at all. On the contrary, his endeavors were admirable. Unfortunately he belongs to a group of people who are full of lymph poisons. Actually, Mr. P. should have let someone else treat him because as soon as the massage began, so many lymph wastes were freed that his body was completely overtaxed. He had to give in to the need to sleep and end the massage. Increasing his intake of fluids might have been helpful.

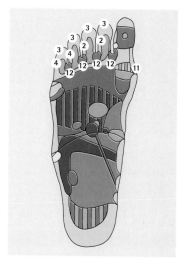

2 eye; 3 forehead, maxillary sinus, and teeth; 4 ear, tonsil, and lateral lymph channels; 11 cervical region of the spine; 12 upper lymph channels

Foot reflexology triggers a process which cleanses the body of its poisons. This frees lymph wastes and washes them out of the body.

When the Body Is Poisoned

In some cases, the body produces a toxin, even though the person has never been seriously ill before. No flu or runny nose makes his or her life miserable, but then a big illness comes along, changing everything.

As absurd as it may sound, small illnesses have a healing effect because they remove poisonous wastes. If that doesn't happen, the body stores them, permitting more serious illnesses. That's how it was with Mr. P. During the next consultation, one week later, he said:

➤ "I'm doing better now. But the eye zone doesn't show any reaction. Instead, the tips of my toes and the liver zone are very sensitive. They become more sensitive every day. Yesterday, I had to leave them out. Strangely, the day before yesterday I caught a cold with a runny nose. I think foot reflexology is damaging me. Now I have even become allergic."

Minor illnesses are helpful because they allow the body to remove poisons. According to our grandparents, a runny nose and cold heal one hundred other illnesses.

Earlier Illnesses Can Play a Role

Answering a question about former liver illnesses, Mr. P. mentioned hepatitis. Additionally, at the age of twenty-five, he had had a serious sinus infection, which the doctor had treated with antibiotics.

Often the liver has a relationship with the eye. The liver is an important organ for detoxifying the body. In the case of Mr. P., it seemed to have been permanently damaged, or at least its function was strongly restricted. I was curious, and so I recommended that Mr. P. have his sinuses X-rayed.

Mr. P. went to get X-rayed. Both maxillary sinuses contained polyps, and the mucus membranes were swollen. The specialist recommended an operation. The next day, Mr. P. found out that the pressure in his eye had risen despite the medications. The doctor told him he needed an operation within two weeks. Despairingly, he came to the next consultation.

➤ "The foot is now so painful at the maxillary sinuses that I cannot touch them at all. The liver zone calmed down a little bit, and I feel better overall. Unfortunately all this did not help, I still must have the operation."

I told him not to give up hope. I also said that I would concur with the idea of operation, but I recommended that he continue his massages and concentrate extra attention on the zones around the maxillary sinuses.

A Dramatic Change

The next consultation showed a completely different picture. The maxillary sinuses were still infected, as they had been for several years, but since the patient did not want to take antibiotics again and he was improving, we substituted simple rinses with salt water. The last test the eye doctor performed before the operation turned out to be a surprise. The eye pressure had improved a little bit again. The eye doctor was glad about the effect of the medications, but he continued to recommend the operation. Mr. P. refused. He wanted to wait a little bit longer. Massages were increasingly pleasant. The sinuses were better, and the infection slowly cleared up. The pressure in the eye dropped so far that the eye doctor canceled the operation and merely continued to prescribe medications.

That is a typical case of how two different events led to an illness. The liver damage decreased the body's ability to detoxify itself, and the sinus infection blocked the circulation of lymph to the eyes. After both illnesses were cured, the eyes recuperated.

Performing foot reflexology is like studying medicine. You get to know the connections, many of which weren't known until recently, even by medical schools.

Please Be Careful!

Of course, you should not just go ahead and use foot reflexology to treat eye illnesses. In cases that are as serious as the example I've described, in which blindness could have been the result, only a very experienced therapist should perform the massage. Under no circumstances should you massage yourself. Not every case of glaucoma reacts so well to foot reflexology. You must always consult an eye doctor.

In Which Cases Can a Massage Help?

Always pay attention to the zone for the cervical portion of the spine because tension there causes many eye problems.

For the following eye illnesses, a massage is worthwhile, and you can use it in addition to medical treatment.

➤ Nearsightedness: If the nearsightedness is not congenital, and is caused by overexertion of the eyes. This is often the case with schoolchildren whose eyes are easily overtaxed. Foot reflexology can loosen the eye muscles and, in some cases, can improve the nearsightedness to some degree.

➤ Farsightedness: When the arms become too short to read the newspaper clearly, we begin talking about farsightedness. This is often a symptom of aging. Here, foot reflexology can be helpful.

➤ Glaucoma: You can use foot reflexology to support medications.

➤ Crossed eyes: For children, being cross-eyed is congenital. It can also be the result of emotional conflicts. During the first years of a child's life, divorce and loud fights between the parents can frighten the child and cause this condition. Foot reflexology helps the child to relax and to trust. However, children under the age of five don't do well with a massage because they are too impatient.

➤ Chronic allergic conjunctivitis: Every form of connective tissue irritation responds to foot reflexology. The massage increases the flow of lymph and the effects of medications.

➤ Inflammation of the iris: You can use foot reflexology to support medication.

Intestinal Illnesses

All the organs in the abdomen, below the stomach, are part of the intestines. People who have never seen an operation involving the small intestine are surprised by the tangle of intestinal loops, which actually are neatly arranged in the abdomen. On the other hand, the colon is arranged relatively simply. It begins at the bottom right in the abdomen, in the vicinity of the groin, and is shaped like a horseshoe, moving through the upper abdomen, finally ending in the anus (see pages 40–41).

In adults, the intestines are about 10 feet (3 m) in length, and the volume is astonishing. The walls of the intestines have many folds. The total inside surface of the intestines is, believe it or not, about the size of a soccer field. This provides space for the intestines to absorb nutrition. In addition, the immune system keeps an eye on what is happening in the intestines, watching what has come into the body from the outside. Unfortunately, as we know, this doesn't provide a secure shield against illnesses of the intestines.

Just as the intestines occupy the bulk of the abdominal area, so they occupy the largest part of the heel of the foot. Just as the different parts of the intestines have different positions in the abdomen, so, for example, the small intestine and the colon have different reflex zones.

When the Intestinal Bacteria Are Disturbed

One could compare the function of the intestines with that of soil. In order for us to thrive, we must absorb nutrients. But without the help of bacteria and fungi, this is only partially possible. In order to absorb the nutrients, certain bacteria and fungi are necessary in the intestines.

Unfortunately, we also eradicate these useful bacteria when we use antibiotics. Many intestinal illnesses which are accompanied by flatulence and diarrhea are caused by damaged bacteria. Frequently, the damage does not occur until months after a treatment with antibiotics. We can often trace the increase of fungi in the intestines, which uses up nutrients and can lead to allergies, back to damage in the immune system of the intestines.

When something disturbs the natural intestinal bacteria, the intestines become vulnerable to germs and fungi from the outside.

The Environment of the Intestinal Zones Is Important

Foot reflexology helps to improve the condition of the intestines, especially if you pay attention to the rule that you must look at the intestinal zone and its environment.

The intestinal zone lies between the center of the foot and the heel (see the diagram on page 53). This zone becomes especially interesting when you realize that disturbances in the intestines can be caused in the stomach, liver, gallbladder, or pancreas. If the digestive juices are flowing too slowly, then you may experience constipation or some other intestinal disturbance. If the bile is not flowing regularly, then you may experience diarrhea. Also nerve-related problems may influence the intestines. For example, some people experience diarrhea when they get excited; other people become constipated when they become excited.

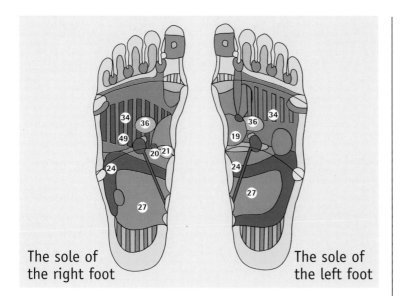

The sole of
the right foot

The sole of
the left foot

19 *stomach and liver, left;*
20 *stomach, exit;*
21 *pancreas;*
24 *transverse colon;* 27 *small
intestine;* 34 *liver;* 36 *solar plexus;*
49 *gallbladder*

The liver zone lies on the right foot around the solar plexus. The gallbladder lies on the right next to the solar plexus point, but somewhat deeper. The pancreas lies about in the middle between the ball of the foot and the heel, but more of it is in the left foot than in the right one, where it only has a small zone.

The Right Massage

Feel the zones in question with the caterpillar grasp and memorize the areas that are pressure sensitive and often disturbed. Don't knead only the intestinal area; you have to carefully incorporate the adjacent zones, too.

Be persistent, but use a light touch. The patient should feel comfortable during the treatment. Each treatment lasts about fifteen to twenty minutes per foot. Patients with acute intestinal inflammation (colitis) should not be massaged in the area of acute pain.

Pay attention to the fact that the feet are pictured as if you had a patient lying in front of you. Therefore, you see the left foot on the right and the right foot on the left.

Disturbances of the Glands

Whenever something does not function right in the body, the cause can be a gland which is responsible for producing the correct level of hormones. Glands have tight connections to the brain, and they are frequently controlled from there. But in addition to being involved with chemical production in the body, glands are subject to emotional processes. Fear, rage, joy, and sadness deeply affect the hormonal balance. On the other hand, balanced hormones produce strength and inner harmony.

Yoga, the Indian art of body control, places a great deal of emphasis on the glands. We also want to work on the glands. I have a short daily program for you which will balance your glandular system with only a few massage grips. The most important glands for foot reflexology are the following:

➢ pituitary gland
➢ thyroid gland
➢ thymus gland
➢ adrenal glands

We generally distinguish between the endocrine glands, which emit their secretion to the outside or into hollow spaces of the body, and exocrine glands, which emit their secretions into the blood or into the lymph.

The Pituitary Gland

The pituitary gland is situated at the base of the midbrain. Important decisions are made at this switch spot. For example, this spot controls the thyroid gland, the hormone production of the adrenal glands, and the production of female and male hormones. No wonder that the pituitary gland is important.

At this point, we want to mention that the proximity of the brain and the teeth can lead to problems with heavy metals, such as mercury, which may be in found in tooth fillings made of amalgam. Unfortunately, the pituitary gland accumulates mercury, which leaches out of the teeth with every bite. Scientists have proved that the pituitary glands of people with many amalgam fillings and dentists who come in contact with mercury show the effects of this heavy metal. Mercury is very poisonous. Therefore, you always need to think about the possibility that this is the cause of an hormonal disturbance.

➢ Mrs. S. was treated for weight gain and a sudden decrease in energy. She suffered from depression and sometimes could not concentrate at all. Since she was overweight, she dieted on and off, but dieting only decreased her weight a few pounds. Of course, the first thought was that she was eating secretly, but that was not the case.

➢ Foot reflexology showed disturbances in the pituitary gland and in the teeth zones. The areas of the teeth were extremely disturbed, showing the cause of the strain. Almost every molar had an amalgam filling. After the patient had the last filling replaced, she felt as if a huge burden had been lifted. The removal of the mercury was supported by foot reflexology.

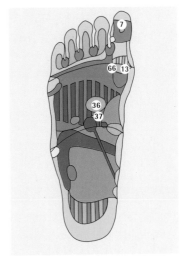

7 pituitary gland; 13 thyroid gland; 36 solar plexus; 37 adrenal glands; 66 thymus gland

Where Is This Wonderful Zone?

The pituitary zone is in the brain area of the big toe, exactly in the middle of the underside (see the diagram on the right). This point is very deep and requires a strong massage. Sometimes at exactly this point, you find warts, fungi, or skin that is scaly. Those symptoms are always a warning that something is amiss with the pituitary gland.

The Thyroid Gland

We know that radioactivity can damage the thyroid gland. After the reactor disaster at Chernobyl in Russia, many people took iodine tablets. Some of those people experienced overactive thyroids.

This gland, which lies on both sides of the larynx, can become a problem without warning. From puberty on, many women suffer from a slight to serious enlargement of the thyroid gland. Normally, except for some difficulty in swallowing, this causes few problems. But when the growth continues and reaches a certain size, we refer to it as a goiter. A goiter is sometimes the result of a lack of iodine. We can prove this with blood tests.

By the time changes show up in the blood, the disturbances in the thyroid gland are dangerous. Then, we see an overactive or underactive thyroid gland. Both need to be treated. In the case of an underactive gland, the body

You can prevent a lack of iodine by using iodized salt to spice your food.

Extreme Mood Swings

In my practice, I noticed a connection between extreme mood swings and the thyroid gland. One patient was so sensitive to iodine and the hormones of the thyroid gland that covering her neck with an ointment that contained iodine led to crying fits. These episodes had no other recognizable cause. Astonishingly, in these patients we found no change in the values for the thyroid gland in the blood.

stores fluid and swells, the eyebrows often fall out at the sides of the temples, and the patient becomes sluggish. In the case of an overactive gland, the metabolism increases so much that the heart begins to race without any reason. This can lead to heart failure. The patient loses too much weight. Both conditions must be treated by a doctor.

Thyroid Problems

Recently, I have observed that more and more patients come in with a strange problem. They have formed antibodies against their own thyroid tissue. The body destroys its gland! In Russia, this kind of illness is a result of damage from radioactivity. Is it possible that other countries have received more radiation than officially determined? Regardless of the cause, in addition to using medication and iodine, you can always treat chronic problems involving the thyroid gland with foot reflexology.

On Top and Below

How can we quickly and easily find the thyroid gland zones in the foot? The thyroid gland is next to the center of the neck; therefore, the reflex zone must lie on the inside of the foot. Since the gland is in the neck area, the reflex zone must be located at the transition from the big toe to the ball of the foot, where we also find the points for the cervical region of the spine. And, in fact, that is where the reflex points are found (see the diagrams on page 55 and at right).

Unfortunately, we cannot comprehend everything that is important during the examination of the thyroid gland. Even with all of our knowledge, we still don't know everything there is to know.

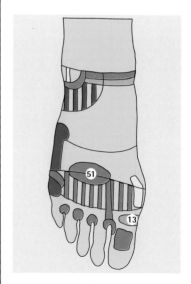

13 thyroid gland; 51 mammary gland

The Right Massage

Knead the thyroid gland points with your thumb every day. I recommend that you do this after you treat the pituitary gland zone because the pituitary controls the thyroid gland.

A Few Remarks About Mercury

Since mercury can disturb the pituitary gland, it can also disturb the thyroid gland. Furthermore, we believe that the so-called hot and cold knots in the thyroid gland usually are related to mercury. Even though we cannot prove this scientifically, I want to call your attention to it. In these cases, foot reflexology helps relieve the suffering.

As you age, a defect of the thymus gland leads to a defect in the body's ability to react to germs.

The Thymus Gland

Many people do not know anything about the thymus gland, and many doctors underestimate its importance because they learned that the gland would lose its function with increasing age. Even though it is true that the gland clearly shrinks from puberty on, the practical successes of thymus treatment suggest that the gland fulfills an important function into old age. The thymus gland lies directly behind the breastbone, below the neck dimple.

According to today's knowledge, its function is to support the white blood cells and to help them defend against bacteria, viruses, and fungi. If the thymus gland can no longer fulfill its purpose, the body loses its resistance, and infections occur.

Then, even though the person has an infection, the body never has a fever or any of the typical signs of an inflammation. The person has a wasting disease, and, at first glance, we aren't able to detect a reason for it. Many older people have this problem. We can learn two things from problems with this gland:

➤ Fever and inflammations are not illnesses. They are the body's healing reactions. We make a mistake when we suppress them, unless they are so strong that they endanger the person.

➤ Many problems associated with aging stem from a weakness in the immune system. The doctor should make an effort to search for the virus and to strengthen the patient's immune system.

We can help the body increase its resistance. The reflex points of the thymus gland lie exactly on the inside of the ball of the foot and at the respective spot on the back of the foot (see the diagrams on pages 55 and 57). You should treat this spot every day.

The Adrenal Glands

You'd never guess from the name that these little glands, which sit on the kidney like a rider on a horse, can cause problems throughout the entire body. Indeed, the adrenal glands control important metabolic and blood circulation functions. These glands are the famous "fight or flight" glands. During stress, they discharge the hormone adrenaline, which dramatically increases circulation. The blood pressure and the pulse also increase. The purpose of this reaction is to prepare the body to fight or to flee. The reaction protects us by warning us that we are in a threatening situation.

In cases of chronic infections and allergies, the thymus gland seems to be disturbed. Therefore, in cases of all of these illnesses, you should treat the thymus gland zone at the same time. Interestingly, almost all patients said that their mood slowly improved with this treatment.

Stress

While once it made sense to run away at the sight of a bear or to swing a club and convince the bear to find something else for dinner, this type of physical aggression is no longer useful. More likely, the "bear" is the driver in front of or behind you on the highway. In addition, westerns and murder movies on TV and at the movies bring the adrenal glands into action.

But too much adrenaline makes us sick, and too much stress produces too much adrenaline. People with high blood pressure should relax, and for that, foot reflexology is wonderfully effective, especially when it includes the adrenal gland zone. This zone lies precisely in the middle of the sole of the foot, somewhat below the solar plexus point (see the diagram on page 55). But be cautious.

➢ Mr. K. was a manager with a blood pressure of 220/120. Medication had lowered it relatively quickly. In addition, Mrs. K. used foot reflexology to help her husband. Unfortunately, she didn't know too much about it. Her treatment consisted of kneading the heart zone and the adrenal gland zone. The massage lasted for fifteen minutes and was extremely painful. During the massage, Mr. K. lost consciousness and woke up in the intensive care unit of the hospital.

This is a typical example of what not to do. Whenever you treat someone, please pay attention to the following rules:

➢ Take your time
➢ Get an overview of the entire foot
➢ Do not cause other people pain
➢ Always treat the entire foot

Be especially careful in case of pain in the adrenal gland zone. Patients should only be treated very lightly. Use stroking rather than deep kneading and use long and gentle strokes rather than short and forceful ones. With these patients, imagine that the object is to allow the patient to fall asleep during the session.

Heart, Circulation, and Blood Pressure Problems

We've already mentioned the important role the adrenal glands can play in cases of high blood pressure. Now, we will look at other reasons for blood pressure changes, and we will learn how to use foot reflexology to reduce the blood pressure.

What Actually Is Normal Blood Pressure?

For those who don't know the meaning of blood pressure values, I want to explain the numbers which indicate blood pressure.

➤ We always state blood pressure values with two numbers, for example, 120/80.

➤ The first value indicates the pressure which the heart and the vessels exert on the blood when they contract.

➤ The second value indicates the tension which remains when the heart and the blood vessels have relaxed.

➤ The tension value is the first number, and the relaxation value is the second number.

Everyone's blood pressure fluctuates. An athlete's blood pressure might be 200/90 during a game. However, during sleep, his blood pressure might sink to 100/70. In order to avoid inconsistencies, be sure that you are using comparable conditions. When you measure your blood pressure, you should:

➤ Always be calm
➤ Use the same arm
➤ Be in the same position
➤ Measure at the same time of day

Don't exercise or eat for at least five minutes before you

High blood pressure is caused by numerous risk factors which you can eliminate, such as obesity, lack of exercise, smoking, alcohol abuse, and stress.

take your blood pressure. Since blood pressure values differ up to ten units, depending on which arm you are using, always measure your blood pressure on the same arm. Also, the difference between sitting, standing, or reclining makes a difference, as does whether you are tense or relaxed. Therefore, always measure your blood pressure in a sitting position when you are as relaxed as possible. In addition, be aware that your blood pressure can be different in the evening than it was in the morning.

➤ If you do everything correctly, values between 110/80 and 130/70 are normal.

➤ People over sixty years of age can have values up to 160/80 once in a while.

➤ Numbers above that are too high (hypertension); numbers below that are too low (hypotension).

Who Determines What Is Normal?

When you compare your blood pressure values, you know where your values fall, whether they are too high, too low, or normal. But who determined these limits? Nature didn't! Establishing specific values is a job for human beings who don't always agree. Therefore, definitions of exactly what is high blood pressure and what is low blood pressure may differ.

➤ Mrs. A. had sudden problems with her circulation. When she stood up and when she stood for a long period of time, she became dizzy and had headaches. Sometimes, she woke up with headaches. The doctor found that her blood pressure was 115/90. However, when he measured her blood pressure while she was standing, her pressure dropped to 90/60. She had a typical case of low blood pressure. She began taking medication, which helped, but when she stopped taking the medication, the problem returned.

Some people only have high blood pressure at the doctor's office because they are afraid.

Hopefully, you already know that I will not advise you to massage this or that zone so that everything will be better. I won't do that under any circumstances because blood pressure fluctuations are a symptom and not an illness. The feet reveal the cause of the disturbance. Therefore, you must look at the entire foot when you want to treat low blood pressure. You should pay special attention to the following zones (see the diagram on the right):

➤ Pituitary gland zone in the middle of the last joint of the big toe

➤ Adrenal gland zone in the center of the foot

➤ Heart zone in the area of the ball of the foot on the inside

➤ Solar plexus zone in the center of the foot

➤ Small intestine zone in the center of the foot and the heel

Low blood pressure frequently occurs in slim people because of a weakness in the small intestine. This is especially true for women. Besides low blood pressure, slim women often also have digestive troubles and constipation. Perhaps the intestinal wastes poison their blood vessels. In women, the zone of the lower abdomen (see page 42) and the pituitary gland are very important.

Trusting the Feeling

My advice is to treat whichever zones you find, even if no doctor supports your idea. For patients who have low blood pressure, you can gradually use a stronger pressure on the sole of the foot over the course of several sessions. This may hurt a bit from time to time. Advise your massage partners to try washing in cold water and then getting back into bed.

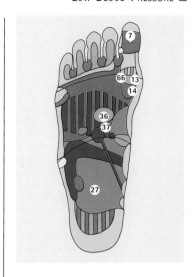

7 pituitary gland; 13 thyroid gland; 14 heart; 27 small intestine; 36 solar plexus; 37 adrenal glands; 66 thymus gland

Pain and sadness are important experiences that you should not suppress or ignore. However, after an appropriate period of mourning, you should look to the future in a positive way and not be dominated by painful memories.

Cold Washing Before Bedtime	
➤ Wet a washcloth with water at room temperature and wash the entire body from top to bottom in just one minute.	➤ Lie down in bed again and cover yourself up to your neck without drying off. Let the warmth of the bed evaporate the water.

High Blood Pressure

Sometimes, you have a difficult time understanding what the symptoms mean in terms of the patient's blood pressure. What at first seems to suggest low blood pressure can turn out to be high blood pressure. The signs can sometimes be similar to those of low blood pressure, as the following case shows.

➤ Mrs. F. sometimes had headaches when she woke up in the morning. While shopping, she suddenly got strong headaches. She went to the pharmacy because she was so dizzy that she was afraid of fainting. Low blood pressure? Actually, when they took her blood pressure at the pharmacy, it was 220/130. High blood pressure! Her doctor confirmed those values.

➤ Mrs. F. was very overweight and was on a diet at the time. She had already lost 22 pounds (10 kg). Why was her blood pressure high at this time? The doctor gave Mrs. F. medication which lowered her blood pressure, but not enough.

She was sent to the hospital. After three weeks in the hospital, her blood pressure values were at an acceptable level again. Mrs. F. continued to diet in the hospital. Her doctors assumed that her high blood pressure was con-

Here's an interesting fact: Vegetarians generally have lower blood pressure than people who eat meat.

nected to her obesity. At the time she was released from the hospital, she was taking five different medications.

Obviously, in this case the high blood pressure was only a symptom of something else. Luckily, Mrs. F. went to a doctor who was able to perform foot reflexology. During the treatment of the soles of her feet, he was able to confirm his suspicion that the problem was caused by an inner poisoning due to the dieting and weight loss.

➤ Her feet were red and sore. They were so painful that a massage was out of the question. The doctor explained his suspicion to Mrs. F. He believed that her body was releasing many poisons because of the reduction of fatty tissue, and these poisons were blocking the metabolism. Her body was suffering from a lack of oxygen, and was trying to make up for the lack by increasing the blood pressure. Thus, the increased blood pressure was the body's attempt to help itself, not an actual illness. Only after a two-week drinking cure, which included water low in salt, did the doctor try foot reflexology again. At that time, he could distinguish the zones for the heart, adrenal glands, and the liver.

Such complicated cases are extremely rare. Nevertheless, this case shows how in foot reflexology, we must keep our eyes on the whole and never be misled by one symptom.

High Blood Pressure Can Have Many Causes

In cases of high blood pressure, you should look closely at the hormonal zones (the pituitary, thyroid, thymus, and adrenal glands). You should also pay attention to the nerve centers in the spine, upper abdomen, and lower abdomen. In addition, pay attention to painful tooth, gallbladder, and kidney points.

Never treat high blood pressure with a strong massage. Only use a soft touch.

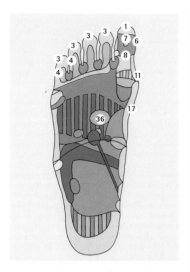

1, 3 teeth; 4 tonsils; 6 cerebrum;
7 pituitary gland; 8 cerebellum;
11 cervical region of the spine;
17 thoracic region of the spine;
36 solar plexus

In modern times, headache and back pain are the two most frequent problems of the adult population. In searching for a cause for his headaches, the patient faces a sea of possibilities.

Headaches

Headaches are one of the most frequent ailments of our time. But all headaches are not created equal. Anything can cause a headache, from simple tension to a brain tumor. Therefore, in cases of chronic headaches, you should go to the doctor for a diagnosis.

➤ Sarah A. had been getting headaches every other day for the last four years. Sometimes they became so severe that she had to stay in bed and could not go to work. She visited a neurologist, an orthopedist, and her internist. All tests were negative. She took medication to be able to go to work. Her family doctor had given up on her. Finally she went to a psychologist to determine whether the cause might be an emotional problem. She was twenty-four years old and without a boyfriend. We might suspect that she had problems relating to people.

As we said, in the case of headaches, all kinds of things can cause them. Therefore, you must remember not to concentrate exclusively on the head zone in the toes (see the diagram on the left).

Tracking Down the Cause

Begin by preparing the feet in order to adjust to their special characteristics. When you then work on the toes, do so carefully and cautiously. These are the smallest zones, and you might miss something if your movements are not cautious.

Begin at the big toe and work slowly to the little toe. Don't forget the sides of the toes, and pay special attention to the back of the toes because that's where the teeth are!

The toes represent different teeth. The big toe represents the front tooth; the second toe, the second and third tooth; the third toe, the fourth and fifth tooth; the fourth toe, the sixth and seventh tooth; and the small toe, the molar and the wisdom tooth.

➤ The patient had a jellylike swelling in the area of both big toes, which were in the pituitary zone. In addition, the sides and backs of the fourth and fifth toes were so sensitive that even the slightest pressure was painful. Also, the transitions from the toes to the foot were very painful.

Teeth Can Be the Culprit

Why do we talk about teeth when we want to treat headaches? Because chronic infections in the head, and especially those involving the teeth, are the cause of many headaches.

Pain in the zones of the teeth can occur in cases of amalgam fillings, cavities, gum infections, and any infections in the area of the teeth, especially those which are not acute and, therefore, are not painful. Problems with crowns and false teeth can also irritate these zones.

Often patients who suffer from headaches have no clue that the source of their sufferings is in their teeth. A visit to the dentist reveals problem areas.

The Tonsils, Another Possible Cause

Next, one often finds inflamed and infected tonsils. The tonsil zone (see the diagram on page 66) is on the fourth toe. We need to remember that people whose tonsils were removed still have partial tonsils because only the palate tonsils are removed. These people still have throat and tongue tonsils (the lymphatic throat ring). Therefore, people whose tonsils were removed can still experience pain in the tonsil zone.

Sinus Irritations

Frequently, the sinus cavities are the cause of headaches. These zones are on the upper side and the underside of the second to the fourth toe (see the diagram on page 66).

➤ The patient was uncomfortable with the zones for the cervical region of the spine and the thoracic region of the spine. The shoulder was especially sensitive, but not as much as the teeth zones. After some stroking, though, she perceived these spots as considerably more pleasant and soothing.

Spinal Problems

The situation at the workplace often leads to tension in the cervical portion of the spine and in the shoulder muscles. In addition, when the eyes are strained, the eye muscles become tense. The entire spine lies on the inner side of the feet, more precisely, at the transition from the sole of the foot to the inside of the foot. The cervical portion of the spine begins at the big toe and ends at the highest part of the ball of the foot. The thoracic region of the spine begins below that (see the diagram on page 66).

All of these may cause headaches that you can relieve via the foot. In addition, infections in the other organs in the head can lead to tensions as well as to lymph strain in the area of the cervical portion of the spine.

A good massage and an attentive masseur can make many an X-ray unnecessary. Remember, you can often diagnose from the feet.

In the middle of the shoulder muscles, you'll find a point that is always hard in cases of such strains. This point is in the middle of the ball of the foot, below the beginning of the third toe.

➤ The chest zone and abdominal zone were fine, except for the stomach and the diaphragm, which the patient perceived as being very painful. The patient confessed that she liked to eat chocolate, but that it did not agree with her. She experienced cravings in the evening, when she felt lonely. Often, violent headaches occurred after that. Red wine did not agree with her, and she had stomach pains.

The Solar Plexus

Frequently, headache patients experience pain in the zone around the solar plexus (see the diagram on page 66) because the center of the body stores all tensions. In cases of chronic pain and emotional problems, breathing often stops unconsciously, and the natural inner massage of each breath does not take place. This blockage occurs almost regularly with headaches. Therefore, massaging this zone helps the lungs unfold properly and dissolves the blockage around the diaphragm.

This zone requires very long and very loving treatment. Under no circumstances should you repeatedly push into this spot with pointy fingernails. Actually it's easy to find the spot because the patient tends to jump off the bed!

Massaging the lower abdominal zone on the inside of the heel brought the problem in her uterus to light. This female patient had a history of painful periods. So we see that the lower abdomen can be another zone of irritation and chronic inflammation (see the diagram on page 70).

Sometimes, the head zone isn't painful, and you can only find disturbances in other zones. Thus, for example, you might find that the regions around the solar plexus are painful.

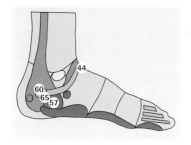

44 groin and fallopian tube;
57 bladder;
60 uterus, prostate, and testicles;
65 male and female genitalia

For women, the cause of headaches and migraines is often found in the area of the lower abdomen. You should always treat these zones.

In addition, strains often lead to headaches and, in women, to migraines.

Many Causes

You see how many connections in the body can be the cause of a simple symptom like a headache. The head zone itself doesn't need to be painful. Sometimes, the only way to determine the cause is to see which zone or zones are painful. Don't be disappointed when you cannot come up with the cause of an ailment in the expected zone. The reason has nothing to do with you or with foot reflexology; the reason is that the connections can be different than you expect.

➤ From massage to massage, the patient perceived the painful zones as being less sensitive. Only the zone of the fifth tooth did not get better. But the headaches themselves had diminished after the fifth session, and she could manage without painkillers. She had stopped eating chocolate. A blood test showed a strong deficiency in magnesium, so she began taking mineral supplements.

On short notice, just before the sixth session, the patient canceled because of violent toothaches. The fifth molar in the lower left jaw was infected to such a degree that it had to be pulled. Unnoticed, an infection had developed at the root of the tooth. Now it had opened up.

From then on, the headaches were gone! The reflex zones showed the connections and causes for the headaches, and the body reacted promptly and lastingly to the massages.

Stomach Pain and Ulcers

Except for a few congenital stomach illnesses, such as excessive acid production, which can lead to stomach ulcers, almost all other stomach ailments are caused by stress or improper nutrition.

You cannot do much with foot reflexology unless you can make it clear to your patient that he has to change his lifestyle. But with a determined patient who is willing to make changes and with foot reflexology, you have a high probability of helping your patient. Certainly massage is a better tool than any kind of acid blocker.

Stomach and Diaphragm

The stomach lies in the center of the body. The abdomen begins where the esophagus enters the stomach. Since the stomach lies directly beneath the diaphragm, it is normally massaged with each breath. When you inhale, your diaphragm compresses the stomach; when you exhale, it releases the stomach. The stomach needs this movement to support digestion. However, people who are under stress often unconsciously stop breathing. The movement of the diaphragm becomes too small, and the stomach doesn't receive the proper massage. This is one way that stress affects the stomach.

In addition, the stress of shock or fear irritates the solar plexus, which controls all of the organs in the upper abdomen. Do you remember the awful feeling in your stomach the last time you were really frightened?

When the intestinal zones react painfully, foreign germs are already in the intestines, and they may have also entered the stomach. Then, with the help of the doctor, you need to sanitize your intestines. You can effectively support this process with foot reflexology.

Don't knead the stomach zone or the solar plexus zone too strongly. While you are massaging those areas, pay close attention to the patient's face. A grimace says more than a thousand words. Many stomach patients tend to overtax themselves, and they rarely talk about their feelings. Therefore, they often say nothing, even when the massage hurts.

How a Stomach Ulcer Develops

Some people are always afraid. Because of their fear, the blood circulation in their stomach changes. Consequently, the stomach produces less mucus to protect the lining of the stomach. This allows stomach acid to attack the cell walls. A stomach ulcer develops. Alcohol and fried foods can damage the lining of the stomach, especially when the diet is low in vitamin C. The result is a chronic infection of the mucous membrane.

The Right Massage

Most of the stomach zone lies on the right foot, in the area where the foot arches (see the diagram below). On the left foot, this area is the liver zone, and only a small bit of it is related to the stomach.

13 thyroid gland and neck;
14 heart, 16 stomach, right;
19 stomach and liver, left;
34 liver; 35 lung; 36 solar plexus
and diaphragm

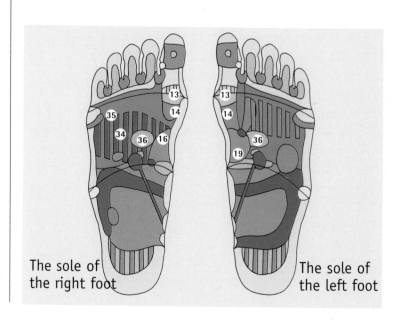

The sole of the right foot

The sole of the left foot

But according to experience, we also need to treat the left foot. The solar plexus point is important on both feet.

Sinus Infections and Sinusitis

Anyone who has ever experienced a sinus infection knows how uncomfortable it can be. The sinuses are normally hollow spaces in the skull. They lie beside and above the nose area. We're not totally clear what their exact purpose is.

When the mucous membranes of the sinuses are infected by viruses or bacteria, they swell. The head feels heavy, the eyes are red, and the nose is stuffy. Sinus infections cause headaches; some can be so strong that the slightest movement produces unbearable pain.

Specialists prescribe bed rest and antibiotics. Sinus infections are dangerous because they can lead to an abscess in the brain. Indeed, sinus infections are no joke.

They are, however, an ailment that responds to foot reflexology. The end joints of the toes are the sinus areas. The areas between the toes are also important because those are the zones which stimulate the head and neck lymph (see the diagram on page 74).

Chronic infections of the mucous membrane of the sinuses can easily occur. Allergies can cause or aggravate the condition. I believe that a large number of damaging substances have a detrimental effect on the mucous membranes. In fact, the cells are so damaged that they become full of holes. These holes allow large particles to enter the bloodstream.

What Happens During Acute Sinusitis?

The mucous membranes swell, and the flow of lymph slows down. The most important thing to do is to clear up the lymph paths again. In addition, you must drink large

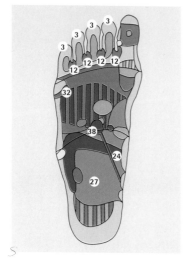

3 teeth and maxillary sinus;
12 lymph zones; 24 intestines;
27 small intestine;
32 shoulder lymphatic ganglions;
38 kidney

Of course, in case of sinusitis, you'll need the appropriate medication in order to prevent an infection. Foot reflexology serves as an additional treatment.

quantities of water. In cases of an acute infection, massage carefully and gently. Under no circumstance should the massage produce pain because pain can produce a cramp, and a cramp slows down the flow of blood, causing blockages.

Massaging Correctly

Begin by stroking the entire foot, from the toes to the shoulder lymph points. These lie at the transition from the toes to the ball of the foot. Treat these lymph zones with small, circular movements. Then, move on to the neck lymph zones, which lie between the toes and go up the back of the foot. The idea behind this order of treatment is that you must first clear the lymph channels. Imagine your sewer line. The water flows from the sink into the drain and then into a big drain pipe. Finally, it flows into a large sewer pipe. If the water stops flowing, the blockage could be at any of those three spots.

During a treatment, we first "free" the large canal, the zones of the shoulder lymph paths; then the smaller ones, those of the neck lymph paths; and finally we work on the zones of the sinus lymph paths themselves. The stream of lymph transports all waste products away with it. Proceed this way for each sinus.

Chronic Infections Can Have...

The situation is completely different when the problem has become chronic. Here's an example of a real case:

➤ Mrs. T. came to see me because she could not get rid of her sinusitis. It began with the flu and high fever. The family doctor prescribed antibiotics. Even though she felt better after a few days, two weeks later, she had a relapse which was worse than the original illness. She consulted a specialist who prescribed another round of antibiotics. This helped, but Mrs. T. had stomach pains and diarrhea from the new antibiotic. Since then, she has had four relapses in three months.

...Completely Different Causes

As always with chronic cases, don't immediately rush to the sinus zones because you could easily overlook other possible causes. The overall picture is always more important than the individual organ.

➤ For Mrs. T., we worked the entire foot up to the intestinal area. We couldn't proceed any farther because that zone was so painful that we could barely touch it. On the other hand, the sinus zones were hardly sensitive at all. At first, therefore, we only worked a little bit around the painful intestinal zone. Within ten minutes, a lively gurgling began in the bowels, which was embarrassing for the patient. After another ten minutes, she began to be restless. She jumped up and went to the bathroom, where she produced a foul-smelling, thin stool.

➤ After two days, the patient called and said that she had experienced diarrhea and stomach cramps since the first massage. At the next treatment, the patient looked as if she were in pain. Her nose was running constantly, and her stomach growled and gurgled. Now it was obvious! First, she had probably gotten an intestinal fungus as a result of the antibiotics. An examination of her stool confirmed this. Second, her body was in the process of helping itself.

While you are taking antibiotics and for some time afterwards, you should make sure that you eat properly and that you drink plenty of fluids.

Getting into the Flow

When something begins to flow, the body has found a way of cleansing itself. Mrs. T.'s body seemed to be trying to cleanse her intestines as well as her sinuses, which were full of fungi. Unfortunately, both are sometimes the consequence of excessive antibiotic treatment. Even though the antibiotics destroy the bacteria, the fungi receive an opportunity to spread. Fungal infections in the sinuses are hard to diagnose, and they are very persistent!

➤ During the second session, the intestinal zone was not as sensitive. The treatment helped it. However, the toes became painful, and the more they were massaged, the more the pain increased. Therefore, we ended the second session with some light strokes to the entire foot.

In fact Mrs. T. improved after the second session. We had told her she couldn't eat sweet food or food containing sugar, and she was also not allowed to drink alcohol. A few days after her stool returned to normal, her sinuses did, too.

> You should never try to achieve anything with force during a massage. Easy, measured applications achieve more. You don't have to stick to a time limit. Pay attention to your patient, and when you have the feeling he or she has had enough, then stop.

Intestines and Sinuses Are Closely Related

During foot reflexology, we often find that both zones are disturbed. The mucous membranes have the same immune system, and as it is below, so it is on top. In chronic cases, always treat the entire foot and the intestinal zones. You may want to include the kidney zone because bacteria often spread into the kidneys, even if the patient doesn't have any symptoms.

Back Pain

Any experienced doctor will be able to confirm that back pains are often the result of problems in other areas of the body. A foot reflexology "scholar" will quickly determine that the spine is often the only place the pain is experienced, the last link in a chain of circumstances. Spinal problems are the most frequent orthopedic illnesses of modern times. The reason is that many of us perform repetitive motions, and most of us do not get enough exercise.

Changing jobs and increasing the amount of exercise are important recommendations which foot reflexology therapists give their patients. The most frequent problems involve the cervical and lumbar areas of the spine. In women, the sacrum and coccyx may also be involved. The pain from these is very similar to the pain of sciatica. We could easily write an entire book about spinal sufferings. However, here we want to limit ourselves to the most important ones because you can get to the bottom of many of the causes during a massage.

The Zones

The spinal zone lies exactly at the transition from the inside of the foot to the bottom of the foot. Since the head has its points in the big toe, we find the cervical portion of the spine at the base of the big toe. From there, the spinal zone runs along the foot to the heel (see the diagram on the right).

The spine consists of thirty-three vertebrae, which are held in place by strong ligaments. However, these ligaments alone are not sufficient to withstand the immense

To treat back pains, you must identify the causes. Shoes that don't fit properly, a lack of movement, physical strains, and even psychic strains can cause back pain.

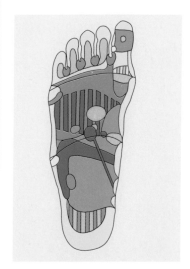

The spine zone runs in a straight line from the top of the big toe to the inside of the heel.

Anyone who has bad back pain knows what it is all about. No one else has any idea!

strains we place on the spine. Many small muscles between the vertebrae absorb the tension. Thus, it is these muscles which produce pain when they are tensed or used improperly. Without the little muscles, the spine would hang loosely on the ligaments. Actually, this is a condition which occurs in cases of complete degeneration of individual sections of the spine. In order to treat the zones of the spine, you must be conscious of the fact that you have to treat the surrounding muscles. Like the hip area, the shoulder area needs thorough attention.

Here You May Use Firmer Pressure

You may treat the spinal zones more firmly. The pressure from the thumb can go deeper. Only by using more pressure can you feel the small muscle zones which reflect the individual spinal muscles.

The Lumbar Region of the Spine

The lowest vertebrae belong to the lumbar region of the spine. We often say that this area is the cross which carries us and which we have to carry.
➤ Constant physical strain and, to a larger degree, emotional tension (especially suppressed rage) lead to a lasting tension in the lumbar region of the spine.
➤ In addition, if the two legs are even slightly different in length, the pelvic area will not be aligned, eventually leading to tension in the entire spine.
➤ Sometimes the small cartilage surface of the pubic bone is injured during childbirth, and the pelvis is no longer stable.

The Right Massage

You need to take into consideration the feet, legs, and pelvic area for all problems in the lumbar region of the spine. Therefore, foot reflexology also includes the zones in the lower leg up to the knee. Interestingly, the foot has no reflex points for itself. You'll have to begin at the highest reflex point of the lower extremity, the knee point on the outside of the lower leg, about the width of four fingers above the outside of the ankle. Feel the entire way on the inside as well as on the outside towards the foot. Problem zones show up as painful areas. Continue on the inside and the outside to the pelvic region, and don't forget the joints (see the diagram below). Only after you have completed the rest of the examination should you check the zones of the lumbar region of the spine (see the diagram on page 77). You should always treat the organs of the pelvis so that you don't overlook the effects of these organs on the spine.

When you have examined the patient, you know what you are going to find, and you can massage the respective zones leisurely. Of course, it is always better to get an overview of all the zones.

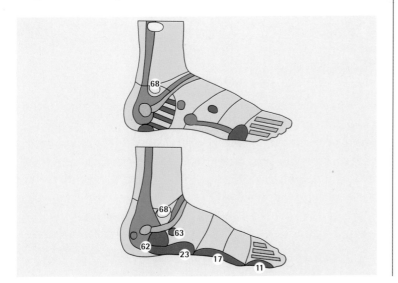

The pelvic zone lies in the area of the lower leg. The reference point for the upper thigh runs up along the lower leg.

11 cervical vertebrae 1–7; 17 thoracic vertebrae 1–12; 23 lumbar vertebrae 1–5; 62 coccyx; 63 sacrum; 68 joints

The Thoracic Region of the Spine

As we mentioned earlier, problems in the pelvic region can affect the entire spine. Therefore, you must also look at the lumbar region of the spine in case of disturbances in the thoracic region. The thoracic region can trigger problems which reach into the chest and abdomen. Throat pains, for example, can be caused by a problem in the chest. Also, aches in the liver and stomach area are sometimes caused by problems in the chest. Foot reflexology can show us exactly where the trouble lies.

Pains in the breastbone are often triggered by something in the chest because the ribs start in the thoracic region of the spine. When the muscular system of the thoracic vertebrae tenses up, the ribs are often blocked, which can trigger pain during breathing. Of course, in such cases, you must examine the lung and heart zones, too.

You may also use relatively strong, deep pressure in the thoracic zone. Strong does not mean rough, but it does mean massaging carefully and deeply.

The Right Massage

All "wear and tear" problems of the thoracic region of the spine can be helped with foot reflexology. If you have found no zones that are disturbed in the rest of the foot, you can strongly knead the zone for the thoracic region of the spine, which runs from inside the ball of the big toe to the inner edge of the foot. In cases where the spine has stiffened because of ossification or degeneration, these treatments are very effective.

The Cervical Portion of the Spine

If only our heads sat directly on our trunks! Although we might have a bit of a problem looking around, we would be spared a large number of neck and shoulder pains.

The cervical portion of the spine is extremely sensitive. The more sensitive and soft it is, the less it is able to endure strains. Car accidents can cause damages that last a lifetime.

The Right Massage

You treat neck pains by massaging the zone for the cervical portion of the spine, the big toe on the inside of the ball of the foot. But don't forget to examine the entire back at the same time. Remember that what is out of order at the bottom, perhaps flat feet, will be out of order at the top, too. Often pain in the neck is not caused by anything in the cervical region of the spine. Instead, it is often the result of a problem in the thoracic region, especially the first and second thoracic vertebrae. Wherever you find zones that are painful or become painful during a massage, that is where the actual disturbance lies, and that is where you must treat the problem. Therefore, don't hesitate to treat the second thoracic vertebra when you find pain in that zone, even though the patient is complaining of pain in the neck. Don't hesitate to treat the eye or jawbone, even though the patient reports neck pain.

That is the real science. Don't let yourself be influenced by seemingly logical information. Only accept what you yourself discover through foot reflexology.

"Sprains" in the cervical region of the spine are a favorite target of over-eager chiropractors who "straighten them out" again. Don't let anyone do that to you. After a period of time, the muscle cramp loosens up all by itself, and the pain decreases. Sometimes, the "straightening out" causes as much lasting damage as a car accident because it can impair the function of the small joints.

Pain in the Lower Abdomen

When we think of pain in the lower abdomen, we usually think of women and their special problems. Actually, in general, women do suffer more frequently from pains in this region than men do. Nevertheless, the reflexology zone is helpful for men's troubles, too.

The Period

The most frequent problems women experience are painful periods. Cramplike pains in the abdomen make the monthly cycle a dubious pleasure. Pains can also occur before, during, or after menstruation. The precise cause of these pains is unclear, but the swollen tissue, a result of hormones, seems to play a role. Additional causes include the relationship a woman has with her own body, whether or not she can let go of her body, and how and why she tenses up.

Many people have speculated that women in developed countries seem to experience menstruation in a different way than women in undeveloped countries, for whom menstruation is supposed to be light and not painful. Still, the fact is that women in all countries endure menstrual pain.

Lifestyle Plays a Role

➢ We were able to determine that women who are vegetarians and who do not smoke have much less menstruation pain than other women.

➢ Office workers suffer more frequently from menstrual problems than women who have a more active lifestyle.

➢ Men have a similar problem. Prostate pains are stronger when a man has a sedentary job.

➢ Emotional problems can occur immediately before menstruation.

➢ Irritation, depression, and aggression may occur frequently.

Luckily, problems in the lower abdomen react quite well to foot reflexology. However, the treatment should start in the middle of the cycle, about fourteen days after the last menstruation. The main zone for lower abdominal pain is not on the sole of the foot, but on the heel, exactly in the hollow below the end of the Achilles' tendon (see the diagram below). This zone is often extremely painful. From the inside and outside of the zone, a band runs over the back of the foot. This represents the groin. These zones are very important. You must always search them for painful areas.

Pain during a period does not represent an isolated illness. However, the hormones involved interfere with the entire body and soul complex. Therefore, you must search for other areas that have problems. Here, the pituitary gland (located exactly in the center of the joint of the big toe) and the thyroid gland (on top of and below the joint of the big toe) can be part of the problem.

The inside and outside of the feet have important reflexology zones. Treat problems in the abdomen gently since the zones are extremely sensitive.

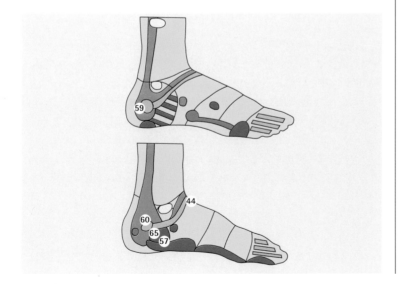

Top: 59 ovaries and testicles

Bottom: 44 fallopian tube;
57 bladder;
60 prostate and uterus; 65 male
and female genitalia

In addition, the nerves in the solar plexus (center of the foot) play a role. You need to feel these points and treat them if they are painful.

We don't want to forget the lumbar region of the spine. Many women suffer from back pains before or after their period. The sacrum region lies at the transition from the sole of the foot to the heel on the inside of the foot.

The Right Massage

If you massage according to the following pattern, you cannot do any harm (see the diagrams following page 11).

➤ Find any painful points. That will help you determine where the main problem lies.

➤ Begin by stroking the sole of the foot. Work the zones of the stomach and lower abdomen easily.

➤ Then, add the hormonal centers, beginning with the pituitary gland. Follow up by working on the thyroid gland, and after that on the glands in the lower abdomen.

➤ Work on all the zones of the lower abdomen, and spend most of your time in that area.

Massage around the painful zones as if you were eating from a hot plate, from the edge in. Only when the center has become less sensitive may you work there.

The entire massage does not need to last more than five to ten minutes for each foot. In case of acute period pains, you should concentrate your massage on the zones for the solar plexus and the uterus. Use light, soft pressure, and work in a circle. When treating lower abdominal pains, you must make sure that you keep the patient's feet warm.

Be careful. During pregnancy, you should avoid having your lower abdominal zones treated since the treatment could lead to premature birth or miscarriage!

Sexual Disturbances

Some women suffer from pains during intercourse; others have difficulty reaching orgasm. (If you want to stimulate your partner, read the chapter "The Erotic Massage.") Most sexual disturbances are based on emotional problems. Many of these are at least partially the result of experiences in childhood or youth. However, some problems can be helped with foot reflexology.

Not Tonight, Honey

Painful intercourse can be caused by an unconscious rejection of sex. Many women feel obligated towards their partner, even though they do not desire sexual intercourse. When this is the case, the body can rebel.

By the way, the truth is that women do not necessarily want to have sexual intercourse every day. The belief that they do was dreamed up by the publishers of men's magazines. The reality is quite different than that portrayed in the magazines. Many woman go through long stretches with no sexual desire at all. This is especially true after they give birth and while they are breast-feeding and raising infants. A lowered sex drive, or even no sex drive, is quite normal.

Listen to your body. If painful intercourse is not the result of giving birth, of an operation, or of an accident, you may need to balance your emotional life, or perhaps you should look for another partner.

Rejecting Old Ideas

We should give up measuring the value of human beings, men and women, by their sex appeal.

Massage Helps

Massaging the entire pelvic region, especially the sacrum and the joint regions, can be very helpful. The vaginal region lies on the inside of the foot about the width of one finger below the ankle. It runs down to the sole of the foot (see the diagram on page 83).

Ailments of Men

In older men, a swollen prostate frequently causes difficulties when urinating. Because the bladder does not empty itself properly, these men urinate more frequently. Often they must get out of bed several times each night.

The Right Massage

The prostate zone lies exactly where the uterus zone is in a woman, directly inside the heel (see the diagram on page 83). A daily massage of this point counteracts a swollen prostate.

When Bacteria Attack

Another male problem is a chronic infection of the testicle. These infections are usually the result of bacteria. Over the years, these bacteria can cause problems, even in other areas of the body. For example, they can interfere with blood circulation and even with blood pressure. Naturally, a doctor should treat this infection with antibiotics, but foot reflexology can accelerate the healing.

In many cases of prostate disturbance, regular exercise can stimulate the flow of blood and reduce the swelling of the prostate.

Sexual Neuroses

I also want to say a few words about men's sexual neuroses. Many men are very sexual beings, as long as women are unreachable or unavailable to them. They have learned that potency equals masculinity, and that influences their feelings of self-worth. Of course, the fact is that potency is a sensitive little plant which easily fades away. Erection disturbances and premature ejaculation are more frequent than you would guess. Men suffer terribly from these problems.

Most sexual disturbances have physical causes that have nothing to do with the penis. Since men have not learned to recognize their own needs and feelings, they also don't feel that anything could be wrong with their self-image. The reality is that many men feel obligated to prove something to a woman instead of opening themselves up to sexuality and tenderness.

Get Rid of Your Prejudices!

An unbelievably large number of men have no sexual desire at all. Did you know that? So, if you suffer from erection disturbances, first check whether you have found the right partner. When you are able to devote yourself to her completely and without any reservations, then she is the right one, and your erection problems will decrease.

The reflexology zone for the penis lies where the vaginal zone is in a woman (see the diagram on page 83), on the inside of the heel, somewhat below and in front of the inside of the ankle. Massage the zone softly and circularly, and stop playing the hero.

Often sexual intercourse resembles dinner. It is a routine that we follow without thinking. But human beings are not machines, and men, too, go through cycles which affect their sexual desire. For days, even weeks, a man can be without interest in sex, and then, suddenly, he has a strong sex drive again.

Toothaches

Teeth seem to be an invention to keep dentists busy. But we need to be aware of the fact that each tooth is embedded in live tissue, and this tissue has enormous regenerative forces. You'll find zones for this tissue on the foot. Of course, foot reflexology cannot fill any holes in the teeth. Clearly, that is a job for a dentist. In addition, the right nutrition and proper tooth hygiene will prevent further problems. But foot reflexology is useful for the following ailments:

➤ Crooked teeth, especially in children
➤ Pains in the upper and lower jaw, when the dentist doesn't find any reason for the pain
➤ Problems with a bridge after having a tooth pulled
➤ Chronic infections of the roots of the tooth
➤ Chronic infection of the mucous membrane in the mouth
➤ Ailments which are caused by the teeth but which are not felt there

The Teeth Zones

We count the teeth from the center. The dividing line is the gap between the two front teeth. The front tooth on the left or on the right is number one. Then, we number them up to the wisdom tooth, which is number eight, all the way back in the jaw.

The first tooth lies on the big toe. The second and third tooth lie on the second toe. The fourth and fifth tooth lie on the third toe. The sixth and seventh tooth are on the fourth toe, and the eighth tooth is on the little toe (see the diagram on page 89).

➤ Mr. G. was twenty-six years old. He was an active athlete who suffered from severe pains in the left knee. They became worse whenever he strained his knee. The sports doctor examined his knee joint, but he didn't find anything wrong in the knee itself, or in the cartilage or the ligaments. He recommended medications for rheumatism. These didn't agree with Mr. G., and he stopped taking them. Injections into his knee joint didn't help him at all.
➤ During foot reflexology, painful zones in the area of the toes of the left foot were found. These pointed to the teeth, especially to the fifth and sixth teeth. This zone lies on the fourth and fifth toe, all the way at the tip. Mr. G. returned to the dentist, who noticed a small infection on an X-ray. The infection was on the fifth tooth on the bottom left. He drilled into the tooth and treated the infection. Mr. G. noticed that his knee pain disappeared as soon as the anesthesia took effect in his mouth. Two days after the treatment, his knee was completely free of pain.

Teeth can be deceptive, as our case history demonstrates. An infection in a tooth caused problems in a joint, even though the patient felt no pain in the tooth itself.

Phantom Pains

Don't be surprised when a zone hurts, even though the corresponding tooth has already been pulled or treated. The nerves in the area of the root of the tooth are usually severed. Even though you don't feel the tooth anymore, the tissue has been seriously disturbed. Whenever a zone becomes painful, something is not right, even if all the dentists in the world say that they cannot discover a cause.

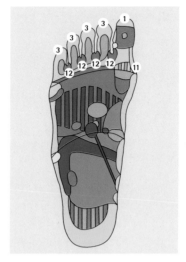

*1 top of the skull; 3 teeth;
11 cervical portion of the spine;
12 lymph zone*

Dentists often do not look beyond the obvious. If they cannot find a cause, they assume the patient is suffering from phantom pains.

89

Nerve Pains

Some toothaches are caused by the nerves rather than by the teeth. The trigeminal nerve runs to the upper and lower jaw. The zone for this nerve is difficult to find. It lies on the inside of the big toe, and it is as little as a pin. When you massage the area, it feels as if little grains of sand were lying beneath the skin. Massage these with a circular pressure until they slowly dissolve.

The Right Massage

Of course, you'll treat the other parts of the toe down to the ball of the foot at the same time you are doing a tooth treatment. This is important because the tooth is surrounded by lymph. In addition, don't underestimate the influence of the cervical portion of the spine (see the diagram on page 89).

Remedy for Crooked Teeth

When a child's teeth grow crooked, you should go to the orthopedist and physical therapist and have his feet checked. Often the child has flat feet or some other problem involving the feet.

A Wise Person Leaves the Wisdom Teeth Alone

Never let yourself be talked into having your wisdom teeth pulled because your teeth are crooked or because your bite is wrong. In all my years of practice, I have not met one patient for whom this procedure straightened the teeth!

Loosening the toes in the morning is an effective exercise to prevent toothaches. Pull your toes a little bit and shake them slightly. That loosens up the tooth joints and affects the zones up to the cervical portion of the spine.

What Not to Treat

Even though foot reflexology is easy to use and is harmless, you should not use it to treat certain conditions and illnesses.

➤ Pregnancy: Treating the lower abdominal zone or the hormonal zone during pregnancy can lead to premature birth or miscarriage.
➤ Skin diseases: You should not use foot reflexology in cases of skin disease on the feet. Massaging the feet can spread germs.
➤ High blood pressure: Do not use foot reflexology in cases of high blood pressure (over 200). The most you should do is to stroke the feet very gently.
➤ Varicose veins: In acute cases of varicose veins and thrombosis of the lower leg, you should not massage the feet.
➤ After fractures: When the leg remains swollen and red after a fracture, you should not massage the leg because the normal function of the nerves is already disturbed.

Foot reflexology is not the right approach for every patient, nor is it the right approach all of the time. Please pay attention to the tips on this page because natural healing therapies can have side effects!

What to Do in Cases of Severe Illness

Of course, when you are dealing with an illness which goes beyond a cold or a runny nose, you must first go to the doctor. However, you won't harm anything by using foot reflexology to get an overview of the situation before or after the visit to the doctor. You can parallel the doctor's treatment with foot reflexology. That way, you cover all bases.

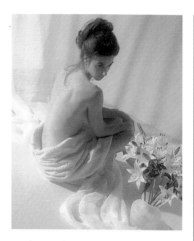

An erotic massage can give your sexual life new energy. Don't be shy!

Unfortunately, we seem to take less and less time in our daily lives to tune in to ourselves, to our partner, and to his or her sexual needs and desires. Eventually, sex, which was once exciting, becomes an obligation.

The Erotic Massage

Even though foot reflexology is primarily a treatment for medical problems, it can also make everyday life nicer because it is so soothing. The Australian aborigines believe, "Paradise is here; there is no beyond." Their meaning is clear. Make everything as beautiful for you as it would be in paradise, and make sure that you are happy and that you make each other happy.

This Is How You Do It

For some people, sex has become boring or routine. Less and less goes on in bed. It is unbelievable what some people come up with when this happens! Some try to rekindle the passion through all sorts of artificial devices. Yet, the answer is so simple. Let sex become a fulfilling experience again. Foot reflexology helps you to do just that.

➤ For a change, turn the TV off and really take time for each other. Turn off your telephone and your beeper. Create a cozy ambiance by turning down the lights.
➤ Lie down on a blanket on the floor or on the bed. You may want some wine to help get started.

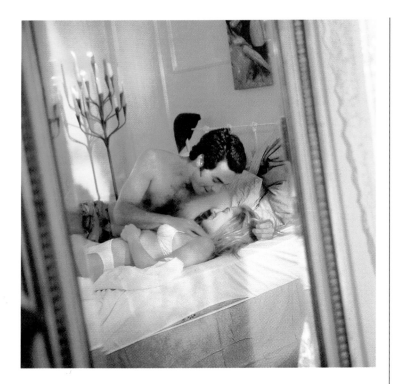

The ambiance should be right during the massage. Try indirect lighting, candles, low music, and some wine to create a relaxed atmosphere.

➢ For this massage you may want to use a little bit of oil. You can add any scent that appeals to you.

➢ Begin the massage by touching your partner's feet very lightly.

➢ Cover the entire foot with oil and loosen up the toes by pulling on them slightly. Of course, you can do this with your mouth, too. You may suck on them very lightly. People from India insist that both partners clean themselves thoroughly before sexual intercourse. This is a nice idea that we can add to our repertoire.

➢ Stroke your fingers alongside the contours of the foot and between the toes. Use the tips of your fingers to circle the back of the foot lightly.

Always put the oil for the massage on your own hands first so that it warms up a little bit. Then, rub your partner with it.

➤ Take one foot in both hands and massage it very lightly with circular movements. Don't forget to massage the zones around the heels! (See the information in the last chapter.)

➤ In some countries, the "feet" include the lower leg, the knees, and the thighs. Stroke the calf and the inside of the lower leg upwards and the outside of the leg downwards. Do that as often and as long as you want, or as long as your partner enjoys it.

➤ Only then should you massage the higher regions. Stroke the insides of the thighs lightly and gently upwards to... No, you cannot touch there yet! Move your fingers very slightly around this area and then take the other foot.

Foot reflexology loosens us up and relaxes us. And, of course, relaxation is a precondition to letting go and enjoying sex.

Have a Lot of Fun

How do you continue? You can probably imagine what happens next. One final tip: If your partner enjoys the massage so much that he or she wants you to continue working on the feet, simply postpone the finale.

Take a small break. Have a little something to eat or drink. Talk for a bit. For a change, let yourself be pampered. You have all the time in the world, because this evening, you are in paradise.

About the Author

Wolfgang Spurzem is an internist and a natural healer with his own practice. Dealing with chronically ill patients encouraged him to incorporate healing procedures outside of classical western medicine.

Dedication

I want to thank everyone who made suggestions and corrections. I especially want to thank my dear wife who stayed up many nights with me and who was able to contribute many good ideas. Also, thanks to my daughter Larissa, who didn't devour all of the pages of the manuscript, but satisfied herself by nibbling on only a few of them.

This book has been carefully written and edited. Nevertheless, neither the author nor the publisher can be held liable for any possible injuries or damages that result from the practical tips made in this book. In the case of serious illness you should, of course, consult a physician.

Picture Source

Bilderberg, Hamburg: 5 (Nomi Baumgartl); The Image Bank, Munich: 16 (Jan Cobb), 92 (Britt Erlanson), U4 (Gio Barto); Tony Stone, Munich: 46 (Chris Craymer), 93 (Timothy Shonnard).

Index

abdomen, lower, 41, 82

acupuncture, 8

adrenaline, 59

allergies, 39

amalgam, 55, 67

appendix, 40

arms, 43

back pain, 77

bladder, 42

blood-pressure, 9, 61

brain, 22

breastbone-spine, 80

breathing, 30, 71

bronchia, 32, 37

colitis, 53

conjunctivitis, 51

diaphragm, 71

ear, inflammations of the middle, 26

esophagus, 37

eyes, 24, 46
  cross-eyed, 50
  farsightedness, 50

foot
  back, 20, 28, 34

ball of the, 29

center, 15, 29, 34, 38

heel, 10, 15, 19, 29, 38, 41

metatarsus, 15, 29, 34, 38

sole, 28

structure, 15

gallbladder, 37, 52

glands, disturbances of the, 54

glaucoma, 46, 50

goiter, 56

Hallux Valgus, 23

hand-rest, 18

headaches, 9, 66

heart, 31

hemorrhoids, 40

holism, 7

hologram, 8

hormone disturbances, 55

inflammations, infections, 39, 73

intestine, 39, 51, 76

joint zones, 43

kidneys, 38, 42, 76

larynx, 32

legs, 44
  lower, 20

liver, 31, 48., 52

longitudinal zones, 7

lung, 31

lymph, 22, 24, 36, 90

mastoid, 23

measles, 26

menstruation pains, 82

mercury, 55, 58

nose, cold/runny, 35

oil
  fragrances, 17, 93
  Jojoba, 17

organs, 22

pain-zones, 21, 27

pancreas, 52

partner massage, 18, 92

pituitary gland, 23, 54, 83

prostate, 42, 82, 86

reflex-zones, 6, 10

relaxation, 45

self-massage, 17

sexual disturbances, 85, 87

shoulders, 9, 34, 36, 43, 69

sinuses, 9, 24, 35, 68, 73

solar plexus, 29, 38, 69, 73, 84

spine, 10, 23, 33, 43, 68, 77

stomach, 32, 52, 71

stress, 39, 59, 71

suprarenal glands, 38, 59

technique
  caterpillar, 20, 23, 41, 53
  massage, 18

teeth, 9, 24., 35, 67, 88

tennis, elbow, 36

throat, 34

thumb, 14, 18, 21

thymus gland, 58

thyroid gland, 31, 33, 36, 56, 83

toes, 10, 19, 22, 27

tonsils, 9,

toxin, flood, 47

ureter, 41

uterus, 42, 84

varicose veins, 17

zone division, 7, 26